STR MANAGEMENT FOR WOMEN

Get Rid of Stress and Anxiety for Life

(Simple Solutions to Start Now to Live a Stress Free Life)

Daniel Lehmann

Published by Tomas Edwards

© **Daniel Lehmann**

All Rights Reserved

Stress Management for Women: Get Rid of Stress and Anxiety for Life (Simple Solutions to Start Now to Live a Stress Free Life)

ISBN 978-1-990268-30-4

Legal & Disclaimer

The information contained in this book is not designed to replace or take the place of any form of medicine or professional medical advice. The information in this book has been provided for educational and entertainment purposes only.

The information contained in this book has been compiled from sources deemed reliable, and it is accurate to the best of the Author's knowledge; however, the Author cannot guarantee its accuracy and validity and cannot be held liable for any errors or omissions. Changes are periodically made to this book. You must consult your doctor or get professional medical advice before using any of the

Table of Contents

Introduction

I want to thank and congratulate you for buying this book.

The book contains proven steps and strategies that will help you manage stress as a way of improving your general well-being. We all know that life becomes unbearable when we allow stress to be in control as it can cripple a person both emotionally and psychologically. This means it is difficult for you to carry on with your daily activities the way you used to, as you are likely to have lost your drive in life. This book is meant to be empowering, as a big part of it makes you aware of the potential you have to conquer stress and other obstacles in life. I hope it will help you gain the knowledge to positively impact your life and the lives of those around you.

The first step towards healing is understanding what stress is, its causes, symptoms, and the effects it may have on your life. This will open you up to the reality of its existence, and most importantly enlighten you on the best approach to take towards managing stress and all of its symptoms. No one deserves to live their lives feeling stressed, as you not only compromise your happiness but also your loved ones. There are many techniques to free yourself from stressful thoughts and feelings and this book is exactly written to help those who may feel stressed and need some practical ways to help deal with it.

It may feel hopeless in the beginning, but once you embark on your journey, one realizes that once they open themselves up by showing willingness and commitment, every other thing flows on its own. The tips and steps to conquering stress are just basic ideas that can easily be instilled in your daily routine. Most of them will focus on changing your thoughts, feelings and approach towards life, aspects that are known to highly contribute to your stress levels. The whole healing process entails letting out negative energy, and learning to be open minded. These are factors that many of us ignore, not knowing the important role they play in determining our general happiness.

The lessons in this book will not eliminate problems and challenges in your life, but will teach you effective and healthy ways to cope with them. It is much about viewing life through different eyes, and not letting any reason to be enough for you to live unhappily. All your worries, fears, regrets and anxiety arise from the mind, and this therefore calls for you to train your mind to be more positive. This is only possible if you are the one in control and not letting it control you. If it is peace and happiness you want, then it is peace and happiness you will get. All you have to do is let this book be your guide through that journey, as each chapter contains helpful information. It is all with the aim of acquiring effective stress management skills through which you end up being healthier, happier and more productive in both your personal and professional life.

Chapter 1: Stress: Causes And Effects

Stress

What is stress? **Psychology Today** defines it as "a reaction to a stimulus that disturbs our physical or mental equilibrium." We all know that stress can take many forms, from difficulties at work to challenges at home. A stressor (why stress happens; the "stimulus" referenced above—anything that causes stress) may be big—you might be in a lot of debt, for example, and have bill collectors hounding your every step. Other stressors may be relatively small— perhaps you are simply caught up in planning a dinner party for a group of friends.

Stress is inevitable—and not only is it unavoidable, it is also necessary. Stress itself is not the enemy. Some stress is good for you, and serves to motivate you to accomplish your goals. Have you ever played a competitive sport, and felt a pressure—accompanied by a strong desire—to beat the other team? Or perhaps when you're at work, you feel fueled by the challenge of tight deadlines and find a thrill in meeting or beating them. These situations also involve stress, but the stress is utilized in a positive way, rather than being allowed to eat at you and bring you down.

No, some stress is good for you. It's when stressors get too numerous or too large in scope or size that trouble crops up—because however large or miniscule the stressors in your own life may be, one thing is for certain: stress adds up. Every single stressor in your life winds up thrown on top of an ever-growing pile where all the various things that stress you out have accumulated. No matter what it is that is causing you the most stress at this current point in your life, it is undoubtedly accompanied by other, smaller sources of stress that lurk in the background of your mind.

The impact of stress

We discussed above why stress happens—but that still leaves the question of what does stress do to us? The answer to that is none too pleasant, as the effects of stress can be extremely detrimental to both your body and your mind. Your well-being can be severely impacted by stress that has built up over time and never been given an outlet. Not only can stress lead to psychological problems like depression and anxiety, it can harm you physically, as well. High stress levels can lead to feeling achy and pained, or simply leave you feeling exhausted and fatigued. Chronic stress is also associated with increases in blood pressure and cardiovascular problems—and these things can have a grave impact on your health. The PsychCentral website provides a list of health problems associated with stress **here**. Although that list is certainly plenty extensive, the sad truth is that it only encompasses a fraction of the ways that stress can negatively impact your health and wellness.

All the stress we feel is a part of the human condition. Everyone, from the smallest child to the wisest elder, is faced with stressful situations on a daily basis. Stress can leave you feeling lost, afraid, filled with self-doubt, helpless and hopeless. You might even feel so burdened by stress that you feel like it has overtaken your life, leaving you with absolutely no control.

The silver lining

The good news is that—in spite of the stress that you find yourself surrounded by on a daily basis—you are not helpless, and there is hope for you. Whether you feel crushed by huge stressors that are beyond your control or simply feel like you are at the end of your rope due to the tedium of daily living, better living is possible.

You wouldn't try to build your dream home without first making sure you had the necessary materials on hand, and the skills needed to use them. Nor should you try to cope with stress without a good set of tools to help you get the results you need—and that is the purpose of this book. I want you to know that you have the power to take the reins of your life in hand, so that you can finally live the life you have always wanted—a life free from the burden of feeling overly stressed. Let me show you the way.

Chapter 2: Causes Of Overthinking

Nowadays, overthinking various life situations and other casual things is an extensive problem. It doesn't imply that educating yourself or thinking over your problems is something terrible, but if you have a habit of twisting whatever around in your head until you see it in every angle and possibility, then you are overthinking. Worrying over different things and events is a natural part of life for lots of people. It usually assists people in finding solutions to their problems and makes them ready to face life challenges and overcome barriers. Just understand that overthinking can happen in numerous situations. Most of the time, nevertheless, you're the one who's triggering yourself to overthink.

Overthinking Can Happen When You Worry Too Much. When you stress, you undoubtedly have a bunch of ideas going through your head continuously. You keep on thinking of the multitude of situations that could happen as the outcome of the circumstance that you're stressing over. Fretting in itself isn't necessarily a bad thing; however,

when it's accompanied by overthinking, you just trigger yourself to experience too much tension.

I think by now all of us know how too much stress can be bad for you. So, by understanding that, you need to decrease those tension levels by worrying less, which will, in turn, prevent you from overthinking. How do you do that?

You can stress less by changing your focus

The fact that you're fretting is because you're afraid that something bad is going to happen. If you're going to think about what will come next, you may as well fill your mind with favorable thoughts rather than negative ones.

You may think that this is simply wishful thinking, but in fact, you can't decide the outcome of every scenario. In the event that an undesirable outcome happens, you can continuously work on altering that result by doing what you believe is needed to do to make it far better. One way or another, what matters is your attitude towards the situation, not the circumstance itself. Overthinking makes you think and feel in extreme ways about a scenario. Shift your viewpoint towards the positive, and you'll overthink no more.

If You are Too Controlling, you Might Be Overthinking. Imposing control upon something or someone is a sure approach to make you overthink. In many cases, you simply have to let things be. If you can't accept that you will continuously over-think things you cannot change.

When you try to enforce control upon somebody else, it could be your ego getting in the way. As I have previously noted in a previous article about becoming less envious, you need to check in with your reasons for doing so and ask yourself if it is due to your ego. If you are struggling with an inflated ego, you desire to enforce control upon everything out of a need for security. It makes you feel like you're not in control when you're in a situation that makes you uneasy. Therefore, your ego starts to panic. Even so, you must work towards finding ease in situations where you cannot have total control.

It may seem like it's just going to make your ego even larger, but in reality, it won't. By getting used to being uneasy, you'll see that the worries you have that triggered you to overthink in the very first place weren't necessary. Not only that, but you'll realize that you were getting in your own way by trying to micromanage the situation.

Overthinking will stop when you get out of your own way. You may not realize this, but often, when you overthink, it's because you are getting in your own way. You need to realize, though, that if you keep getting in your own way by overthinking, nothing will improve. Things will ONLY get better when you take action for them to do so.

By the way, if you're questioning why some people have an inflated ego, simply understand that there can be numerous reasons that they do. It could be due to low self-esteem or low self-confidence. Having a poor view of yourself might lead you to overthink.

You View Yourself Poorly Which Causes You To Overthink:

You're bound to think too much about certain things when you have low self-confidence or low self-esteem. If you have low self-esteem, you'll keep thinking about how other individuals see you. You'll likewise tend to be more critical of yourself since you'll believe that you're not as worthwhile as other individuals. The same is true for issues of low self-confidence.

Whenever you're confronted with a difficulty, you won't feel capable of being able to overcome it. You'll state to yourself that you're not good enough for this or for that. And you'll find all the reasons you can to escape from your issues. In truth, though, you'll, once again, get in your own way by making yourself think that you're unsatisfactory to accomplish something. But you will never know whether or not you're good enough if you do not try. It's just by doing something that you'll see that you can do it.

Yet, the act of simply thinking about these things will lead you to overthink as they tend to make you worry. In my first point, I discussed why stressing can make you overthink and what to do about it. One excellent way to do this is by doing what you're intimidated or afraid to do.

If you do not go beyond today's version of yourself, you will never evolve into a better more evolved version of yourself. To be able to do this, you must to let go of the old version of who are, the one that is terrified venturing into the unknown. It's only by leaving the safety of your comfort zone that your confidence will grow, and trust me, it will grow exponentially when you face your fears and venture out of your comfort zone! As your confidence grows, so will your self-esteem considering that you'll see that you're somebody who's good enough to do something you once believed you were not capable of doing.

You're Not Living In The Present Moment.

When you're not conscious of the present moment, you get lost in the never-ending sea of your ideas. As I've discussed previously, you wind up creating all sorts of scenarios in your mind. However, if you work hard to deliberately remain conscious of the present moment, you can solve this conundrum.

To do this, you simply must start to practice mindfulness. Mindfulness is the state of being in the present moment, by concentrating on what's going on around you and within you in the present moment. You just live in today, in this minute, this moment.

Release your worries and concentrate on what is right in front of you. When you achieve mindfulness, you understand that the present is the only truth there is. You likewise recognize that the past is already gone, and the future has yet to occur. By understanding that, it becomes apparent that the only time you can alter your perspective is the NOW, not the past or the future, but this very moment. You must live in the now in order to stop overthinking about what may or may not happen tomorrow. That's why being mindful of the now can assist you to stop overthinking. Not only that, but it also assists you in letting go of unfavorable ideas.

As soon as you've let go of negative thoughts, you will enjoy peace of mind. If you have too much tension due to overthinking, then you need to work on lowering that stress. Or you can work on reducing your tension levels if you feel like your stress is what's causing you to overthink.

Due To The Fact That You're Rejecting Reality, You're Overthinking.

As I've said in my point about micro-managing things, you can't manage every single aspect of your life. Some things will have results that you cannot control, no matter how much you wish you could. That's why it's essential for you to accept that some things are just the way they are.

Sometimes, you just have to let things be.

It's futile to drive yourself crazy overthinking about the bad just because of how it makes you feel. Even if you think about it all day and night, it won't accomplish anything other than making you worried. Accept that the bad will sometimes happen to us all.

Most things never go 100% according to plan. And yes, sometimes, bad things take place. You must not lose hope just because something bad occurs to you or to someone you care for. If you never had to deal with any difficulty, there would be zero space for growth. That's why it's important we experience the bad and the good in life - so we can grow, evolve and become better versions of self.

Chapter 3: Powerful Guidelines On How

To Deal With Stress

The acquirement of knowledge on how to deal with stress and applying stress management methods are becoming even more important, due to the fact that stress has become an integral component of our daily lives.

Nowadays, it is totally normal to be stressed and under mental as well as physical pressure in our personal and professional life. The majority of people haven't even figured out effective stress management methods.

Being extraordinary busy and working long hours has become trendy, but have you known the negative influence that this high tautness can have on your life? Firstly, you should be aware that our bodies are not prepared to face constant stress periods day after day.

Therefore we need to make sure to find intelligent solutions on how to deal with stress and find stress management methods that allow us to deal with pressure in form of worries as well as physical and mental pressure.

This helps us to prevent typical afflictions that were affected from permanent stress, such as depressions, chronic fatigue, heart diseases, sleeping problems and terrible migraines.

How to deal with stress? In the following you will find some really amazing guidelines and stress management methods that help to deal with stress in order to reduce and finally avoid all kinds of tensions.

What is stressing you? Before you can begin to combat your burden by adapting stress management methods, you'll need to know exactly what is causing your mental pressure.

You could start some kind of a stress diary where you note every aspect in your daily life that has caused trouble, worries, stress and pressure. The more accurate you identify patterns that are causing tensions, the more successful you will be dealing with stress.

Declare the war against stress. Once you figured out the causes of your tautness you can implement stress management methods to prevent these. Integrate such an easy method as to calm yourself down. Breathe in deeply and try to analyze a specific situation as antiseptic as possible, whenever you face stressful situations.

(Note that emotions are causing stress, therefore we focus on a businesslike analysis without emotions). Another very powerful technique on dealing with stress is to be prepared for stressful situations. Always have a contingency plan prepared for these circumstances as well as unexpected events.

The efficiency of such a plan is that it enables you to react properly in these situations, without the necessity of feeling pressured at all, since you have outlined procedures for stressful eventualities.

Develop a compensation for stress. The implementation of activities that help to reduce stress is very powerful when dealing with stress. Compensate stress by exercising regularly, taking a stroll in the park, listening to relaxing music and similar things that allow you to ease off.

Face your problems. A lot of pressure and tension will be reduced when starting to face the origins of these worries. The attempt to escape from these issues will not help you to reduce stress, but instead cause a lot more tension. The attempt to run away from problems is very unproductive when dealing with stress.

Replace stress with positive emotions. There is absolutely no necessity to feel pressured in situations that can´t be changed (like getting stuck in traffic).

If you have come to the decision that a specific situation can´t be changed currently you should actively try to replace the pressure with positive emotions. You could turn on the radio with your favorite music and relax, while being in a traffic jam.

The willingness to implement stress relieving techniques is the first and most important step to create a lifestyle without pressures. Stress management will certainly require some discipline and effort, but it will enrich your life.

To be precise: knowing how to deal with stress by applying stress management methods will help you to cope with a lot more difficult situations and improve your personal development.

Chapter 4: Internal Stress:

Internal stress is nothing but mental stress. It is induced in a person when he over thinks or over analyses. It is also introduced when something keeps bothering a person to no end.

Environmental Stress:

This kind of stress is caused by external factors, i.e. factors other than one's mind. It could be someone's remark, or a calamity.

Biotic Stress:

Those forms of stress that are environmentally caused and are naturally existent are called Biotic Stress forms. For example, too much of wind may cause trees in a particular area to be uprooted. Excessive sunlight may cause drought or even lead to the formation of a temporary desert. Such forms of environmental stresses are called biotic stresses.

Abiotic Stress:

This form of stress occurs when non-living factors cause stress in living beings in a specific environment. The variable which is non-living in nature must effect the environment to such an extent that it should in turn effect the living population in the specified area.

Chronis Stress:

Chronic stress is nothing but reaction of a human mind to prolonged exposure to mental pressure. It is different from normal stress in the sense that chronic stress occurs after a long period of exposure while normal stress induces immediate reactions too.

Occupational Stress:

When a person suffers from stress due to issues arising out of his occupation, it's known as occupational stress.

Traumatic Stress:

It is an extreme form of stress that effects people till they break down emotionally. It involves the introduction of anxiety and depression in their extremes. Usually referred to as deadly, this form of stress can prove really push a person towards a mental black pit. There are little chances of recovery from such pits.

Stress, as we witnessed in this chapter is wide-ranging and many-faced. It is primarily mental in nature but can spread its wings to other aspects too. Let's move on to the next chapter which will focus on what factors are responsible for the causing of stress in your lives.

What Causes Stress?

Anything that causes stress is called a Stressor. It can be better defined as an experience, event or inducer that causes or sets the tone for the introduction of stress in an individual. Stressors are therefore, basically those causes that are responsible for happening of stress in individuals.

Some of the most common factors have been enlisted below:

Life events

Some of our life experiences leave behind a greater impression on our minds than others. Some of such experiences have so much of gravity attached to them that it becomes next to impossible to simply forget them.

It becomes a daunting task to fight back the tears thinking about how you were sexually assaulted when you were twelve. You cannot wipe the memory of when your dad passed away when you were still in school. It is not a cakewalk to simply stop recalling all those times you were subjected to bullying in your high school.

The kinds of events we are talking about are nothing depressing per se but are really important to you. They could be the birth of a child, the demise of an already ailing dear one, introduction to hostel life, graduation or having sexual intercourse for the first time.

These sorts of life events needn't necessarily be gloomy or sad. They could have the capability to induce the brightest of joys in one's life. But when these events do not go as planned, or something distasteful happens during the occurrence of such events, it leads to the causing of stress. The importance these events have in your life is so crucial that a slight change directing the event towards an undesirable result could become a cause of stress.

Bad experiences

Not everything that happens in our lives is rosy and rainbow inspiring. It is a given that life is ready to hand you out lemons at every twist and turn. Despite your care and caution, mishaps and accidents are bound to occur. You cannot escape the harsh reality of life- it'll screw you over. You cannot prevent that. But what you can do is prepare yourself for stress. The next chapter will deal with how to do it,

Crises

Crises are those events that happen without a notice. They are unpredictable and can rarely be foretold about. They arrive with a gush of wind and leave without a trace. They catch you off guard and shock you within seconds. Crises happen all the time, with everyone.

An earthquake or a tsunami could classify as a crisis. In order to qualify as a crisis, an event must be unforeseen and unpredictable. It should come as quick as a fox and leave as fast as an arrow.

Crisis situations are extreme in nature. Their effects are far ranging are not temporary in nature. They completely toss normalcy to the winds and create whirlwinds of worries. A string of such worries causes what we know as stress. Urgent circumstances like an accident is one example of crisis.

Daily life nuisances

Your everyday life is full of minor and simple events and things that cause you mild annoyance, disturbance and diversion of attention from things that are more important. No one leads a perfect day. There will be at least one moment in a day when things don't go our way. Such moments are common causes of stress.

Work related stress is the most known form under this category. Office environments are turning more competitive by the day. The corporate circles are going for people who can work like machines and give out results within the blink of an eye. Amidst such a scenario, it is nothing but natural that tensions and minor hassles are bound to arise.

Household is another area where stress pops out its ugly head. Be it the annoying neighbor who doesn't shy away from eavesdropping on you, or the milkman who doesn't come in time thereby causing your kids to miss their breakfast milk; stress is present in the household scene as much as it is in the office surrounding.

Academic stress, though is desirable, when taken in huge amounts may lead up to a negative impact on the young minds. It is desirable that a little bit of stress be applied on the academically engaged minds. However, when these mild pressures turn into humongous ones, it backfires and turns ugly.

Miscellaneous forms of stress can be stumbled upon during an average day of our lives. The taxi driver not agreeing to a payable sum of money, your boss not being satisfied with your work, your co-employees talking behind your back, your kids not performing good in their studies, your husband coming home late from 'work'; the degree and frequency of stress may differ, but its presence cannot be denied in our daily life. In this form or that, it stays and feeds off us.

It eats away our mental peace bit by bit without us noticing any difference. It arrives as a bother, turns into a worry and transforms into stress within a matter of seconds. Learn to stop this from happening by adopting some very basic tricks. The next chapter will guide you to a stressful life.

Chapter 5: Avoiding Extreme Distress

"Being busy does not always mean real work. The object of all work is production or accomplishment and to either of these ends there must be forethought, system, planning, intelligence, and honest purpose, as well as perspiration. Seeming to do is not doing."

Thomas Edison

One way to manage your stress levels is to setup a system which helps you avoid extreme distress altogether. Note again that stress is not always bad, so you don't want to avoid all kinds of stress all the time. A bit of adrenaline in your system when you are confronted with new situations is a natural way for your body to deal with novel situations. What you want is to prevent the stress from becoming unproductive and paralysing.

Avoiding extreme stress needs the correct mentality. Our brains are quite powerful in solving problems, though they must be given the right problems to solve. Hence, managing stress is a mentality to a large extent. If you have the right state of mind, you already have setup defence mechanisms to respond to a variety of stressors that may affect you during the course of a day.

If you ask the right questions, the brain is very good at delivering the right answers. However, it is all too easy to ask wrong questions and end up nowhere. Examples of wrong questions are as follows:

Why is it always me who has to do everything?

Why is everything failing today?

Why can I never become good at this?

How come of all the people, it should be me who has to suffer like this?

Why people are so dumb? Do I have to tell them everything?

Why did I get myself into this mess?

Why can't I learn this/do this/memorise this like everyone else?

Instead of asking these negative questions which will only make you feel worst about yourself and certainly does not help the situation you are in, you can ask yourself positive questions focused on solving the problem as you saw earlier in the exercise.

Anticipate Stress

Naturally, a way to avoid and manage extreme stress is to setup defences long before you get there. Most people find two main areas as the chief source of stress; scheduling issues and dealing with people. Combating these two sources needs effective time management and good assertiveness skills so you can deal with people without getting too emotionally stressed. These two anticipation strategies are explained below.

Time Management

Time management is an extended topic and a separate course on its own.

However, it is important to know the link between good planning, scheduling and anticipating stressful situations and managing stress.

The following tips help you to quickly review the way you manage your time and take steps to reduce your stress levels by anticipating them or by making yourself more productive. After all, if you have more time available, you are much less likely to get dangerously stressed.

Anticipate stress based on time of occurrence. Use your daily log to spot patterns of stress. Is there a particular time of day/week/month/year that you are more stressed than others? Are you happy with this stress level? If not, how can you spread your tasks in order to stay in eustress zone?

Have a Mission Statement. Knowing what you want from life and when, enables you to choose your tasks based on your priorities, manage your time better and reduce your stress levels. A Mission

Statement defines your life's purpose and achievements; this is what you want to leave as your legacy. Hence, you need to spend a fair amount of time formulating and updating this over time to make sure you will get where you want to be eventually.

Be Happy Busy. You can either be unhappy about the lack of time and blame everything for it, or you can choose to be a happy busy person who takes the lack of time as a challenge. This is only a mentality, so you can easily choose the right mentality and get all the benefits, or just be unhappy. It's up to you.

Use weekly reviews. Take steps to monitor the level of your workload against the time you have available. You can achieve this by weekly reviews. Use this time to plan for the activities of the coming week and also check last week's ongoing events to spot trends which can help you in anticipating and preparing for future events.

Learn how to anticipate and predict. Using dead time is a great way to add time to your life. Time is money, there is only so much you have and every little you save is for you to spend. If you anticipate the dead time event (such as sitting in Dentist's waiting room) or predict it accurately (by taking an article to read in what you think is 10 minutes wait) you can easily reduce your stress level. You will no longer feel the pressure from standing in a queue or getting stuck in traffic, because you have taken steps to use that time to its fullest extent.

Use structured planning. Plan everything, starting with the purpose. Planning is not about organising and scheduling, it is more about knowing what you want to achieve, why you want to achieve it and when and understand what problems may affect your plan. If you know these, the scheduling part is the easiest part.

Offload to calendar. If you think you are not organised, then research time management models to devise a system that works for you. Use a system that can take care of your daily errands easily and free your mind from little worries. The less you have to worry, the less stressed you are. Off load this worry to a calendar system you can rely on. Remember, worries can accumulate in your head and push you towards the distress zone.

Tips on Time Management

- Use a consistent knowledge management system, where you know exactly where a new piece of information goes. For example, set a mind map, or a use notes in Outlook, or Word document or whatever works for you as long as you know in two seconds where you should put a new piece of information, whatever that may be.
- Use the two minute rule advocated by David Allen. If an action takes less than two minutes, do it there and then. There is no point keeping it around and coming back to it later because the overhead is longer than actually doing the task. This saves a lot of time.
- If you don't have to do it then don't do it. Sounds really simple and obvious but just about everyone falls into the trap of spending time on unimportant things and only realising at the end that nothing would have changed if they haven't spent time on it. One less task to do means you have more time to spend on important tasks.
- Sync all your emails, tasks, contacts and your entire settings and files across all your devices (home computer, mobile, work computer, laptop and so on) so when you change something you let the machines take care of the rest.
- Set up automatic actions based on emails. For example, if you ordered something from Amazon and got a confirmation email, use that to create an action automatically scheduled for seven days later to remind you to check if the parcel has been delivered. The more you offload from your mind to machines the more you can think of other things.
- Set up automatic reminders for yourself. In other words, get the machines to check on you. For example, use a periodic reminder that comes up on a regular basis to remind you of this "Are you inventing things to do to avoid the important task?" This simple message will help you to evaluate your actions and get back to the real work.

Dealing with People

Apart from the lack of time management, the other major source of stress is dealing with people. This can become a major source of stress for some people. This topic is equally vast as handling people and interactions is an essential skill in both

39

our personal and professional lives. Certain aspects of people management are more important in dealing with stress and recognising such areas allow you to anticipate and manage your stress levels more effectively. The following are the key areas in dealing with others:

Interruptions. Interruptions especially when you are busy with an important task, are often distracting and a source of irritation. They can affect your performance and put you under unnecessary pressure. Such pressure is very distressing and therefore unproductive. There are a number of simple techniques which you can use in reducing such interruptions, for example you can setup a system which only allows others to interrupt you at certain times of the day. You can turn off your email notifications and only read your emails at lunch time and won't get interrupted when you are in the middle of something else.

Saying NO. Being able to say No is critical. If you don't say no at the right time, you may be taken advantage of or be treated unfairly. This easily creates anxiety and lead to extreme distress. By saying No, you also show people, including your boss, that you can stand firm in the face of opposition and defend your own position which is of course a critical quality to have.

Delegation. Knowing how to delegate to others is an essential skill to reduce stress levels. Many stressors are the result of been overwhelmed with high levels of work, over estimating one's own abilities and the need to achieve perfection. Delegation is a great skill to rescue yourself from dangerously high levels of work, while also empowering others and expanding your reach and throughput.

Assertiveness. When dealing with others, you can appear to be aggressive, passive or assertive. An assertive behaviour is critical in reducing stress levels while making sure you get what you deserve. This is explained in more detail below.

Assertiveness

Maintain Your Balance

- Balance your work with leisure and exercises.
- Develop hobbies, a variety of interests and activities. Have on-going projects that calm you and focus your mind on something completely different.
- Don't keep your problems to yourself. Reduce your anxiety and anger by sharing it with others. If you don't want to share with your friends and family, share them anonymously on the internet with many other likeminded and helpful citizens of this planet.
- Develop relationships and engage in social activities. Life is not about projects, it is about people.
- Don't expect the world from yourself. Set specific, measurable, achievable and realistic goals and stick to them.
- Learn to accept what cannot be changed.
- Sometimes give in to a change request, even if you think you are right. It's not always worth it!

Aggressive behaviour, as the name suggests, is about being demanding and uncompromising. Such behaviour can create an atmosphere of mistrust and have negative effect on your emotions. Being aggressive to others can easily lead to stress as you are aroused either by your own behaviour or as a result of the reaction you receive from others. In contrast, passive behaviour is to accept the situation and not confront it at all. Indeed, this behaviour may lead to a lot of stress as you regret accepting more work or responsibility that you can handle. The correct approach is to use an assertive communication where you express your needs without jeopardising your position or appearing aggressive to the other person. You want to be firm but fair in achieving your goal and defending your position without getting emotional. The best way to understand an assertive behaviour is to compare its qualities with the other two approaches. These are presented below.

Posture

Aggressive. Dominating posture, upright standing, hands can be on hips, feet firmly apart, movement can be erratic, uses pacing, try to show domination through physically prowess

Passive. Head down, appear small, sitting when the other person is standing, sloppy-shouldered

Assertive. Upright, firm but relaxed, evenly balanced, reasonable distance from the other person (based on culture)

Content of speech

Aggressive. Threatening, demanding, bickering, extreme points of view, excessive exaggeration, blaming, uncompromising, attacking personality, pushy, bossy, ordering others what to do, deciding for others what to do

Passive. Lots of "I'm sorry" in conversations, mumbling, avoiding, changing subjects, lots of sighs and sense of hopelessness in the speech, accepting their faults easily, bringing themselves down, not stating what they want, dismissing own benefit for the benefit of the other, avoiding confrontation, accepting jobs without negotiation

Assertive. Fair and logical, lots of explanation backed with facts, gives praise and criticism systematically, not afraid to say 'No', willing to receive constructive feedback, state what they want firmly, clearly and kindly, understand what they and others are entitled to, willing to stand up for anyone to maintain fairness

Timing

Aggressive. No respect for other people's time, interrupt others in mid conversation, talk loud & don't let others talk

Passive. Quiet, hesitates to state comments, has many gaps where others come to cut in

Assertive. Giving equal time to all views, taking charge to make sure all parties are heard, asking all to agree to a system where everyone can talk and expect to be heard

Eye contact

Aggressive. Staring, direct gaze, looking down on people, glaring, maintaining eye contact for longer than normally expected

Passive. Avoiding eye contact, looking up form a lower position (such as a child to a parent)

Assertive. Relaxed gaze, attentive and gentle, looking at the same eye level

Voice, tone, volume, etc.

Aggressive. Loud, threatening, non-stop, aggressive

Passive. Quiet, childlike

Assertive: Relaxed, firm, gentle, nice on ears, medium volume

Facial expression

Aggressive. Clenched teeth, eyes rolling, angry, intense, mean trouble

Passive. Guilty, apologetic, sad, blank look, nervous smile

Assertive. Relaxed, supportive, firm, pleasant to look at.

Gestures

Aggressive. Animated gestures, pointing, aggressive poking with finger, clenched fist, crushing handshakes

Passive. Hands and arms on sides, nervous fiddling, defensive position such as crossed arms or crossed legs

Assertive. Open and relaxed gestures, gestures used to emphasize points

Tips on Managing Stress Levels

- *Have a positive attitude.* If you accept that sometimes stress is beneficial, you will get fewer side-effects.
- *Anticipate stress.* Discuss situations where you think you might be stressed when dealing with your family, friends or colleagues. Working together can greatly reduce your stress level having known that you have done something about it.
- *Clarify responsibility.* If others know what is expected of them and you know what is expected of you, you can substantially reduce stress as a result of miscommunication or lack of clarity. Be open to issues and expect that their occurrence is a natural part of your progress and learn how to handle them efficiently.
- *Learn to relax.* When you are in the middle of a situation, you may find it difficult to get out, but indeed even taking a few minutes to calm down by sitting on a comfortable chair, breathing deeply, doing yoga moves or listening to music can do wonders. Taking a shower, massage, meditation and systematic relaxation techniques can help you to bring your emotional state to a neutral level and effectively put yourself in the eustress zone again.

47

Chapter 6: Social Media & Stress

We have all heard of outlets such as twitter, Facebook, and MySpace, just to name a few. Social media can be fun and useful, but only in moderation. Essentially, the purpose of social media is to connect and bring people together, without having to be on the phone or in purpose with them. Whether you post pictures, videos, status updates, or tweet, it is all social media. While is all sounds fun and good, there are most definitely positive and negative effects in regards to social media.

Before we delve into the negatives, let's start with a few positive attributes that social media can sustain. First and most obvious, social media allows people to stay in touch over long distances. You no longer have to call or text someone to connect with them, in fact, with the click of a button; you can reach hundreds of your followers/friends. This concept allows information to be spread extremely fast, and can be shared at lightning speeds. Ever heard of the "fact" that humans eat an average of eight spiders during their sleep in a lifetime? Well, this "fact" was made up to prove how fast trivia spreads on the internet.

Is technology the savior of business people or the bane of their existence? Stress in business is as old as business itself. In modern times, a number of technological devices have appeared to make business more efficient and more productive. These devices include computers, cell phones, and Blackberries. Each device helps organized data, maintain communications, and facilitate business functions. In theory, this should reduce stress in the workplace but in reality, these devices have created new or different workplace stress factors. This is a trend in business that is not likely to   change.
 Stress in the workplace is not a new concept. People have always worked long days, under difficult conditions. There used to be no healthcare, no workers

unions, and competition was arguably fiercer than it used to be. Yet, the employee of today often has difficulty dealing with stress and its symptoms. Many stress factors that have existed for decades are still prevalent today.

Cell phones, computers, texting, voice calls, among others, are all new outlets of stress. Does technology help us reduce or promote stress? The people that believe technology is a negative in society and needs to be abolished are now the extreme minority in the modern world. Everyone would rather believe that devices will help deal with all the clutter and stress of their everyday lives. As time progresses, people expect more and more out of technology. This leads to new and sometimes futuristic features that amaze many of us. Workplace technology feeds off of this mentality, and continues to advance.

Businesses used to deal with mounds of papers and physical documents, and would have to hire secretaries and data entry specialists to manage it all. Computers soon arrived, and changed the entire professional world. It became possible to globally compete and keep track of other companies' activities on a minute-by-minute basis. Global competition became a huge source of stress, because the entire world became involved in every decision made. Employees' modern fear of job loss is directly tied to technology in the professional workplace.

Never before have we witnessed such an influx of offshore job replacements and companies struggling to find the fastest and cheapest way to produce their products. The average, everyday employee has to take care of themselves and possibly a family. It is near impossible to compete with the wages of Asian and Indian workers, as even if you were able to work for such low wages, the majority of countries have laws prohibiting people for working with such low pay.

The cell phone has become a necessity in a very short period of time. It is considered so important, that the United States government will even supply a phone to the poorest of citizens. Pick a person off the street, 99 times out of 100 they will have a cell phone. Looking at the surface, cell phones are an extremely beneficial invention. When off work, business people used to be completely cut off from their jobs and projects. The cell phone introduced a new type of stress for all professionals, because not only did they have to deal with problems at work, there is now no excuse not to do work when not in the office. For only about ten dollars a month, it is an oddity when the modern businessperson does not own a cell phone. It is only natural to assume that people who own cell phones will greatly increase productivity and accessibility. As we have discussed, this is not exactly what will happen. Cell phones enable professionals and all people to stay connected with each other 24 hours a day, every day. Doing so disallows people to have true personal lives, and to separate professional and personal. Just because you are not in the office does not mean you cannot call your boss or keep up with projects. The workplace is no longer an escape from personal stress and home is no longer an escape from professional stress.

Cell phones are inarguably the largest stress producer in the workplace. Walk down the streets of any city and you will find multitudes of businesspeople using their phones at work, in the car, or while walking. It is possible to use a cell phone silently and without speaking, so they become an easy distraction for many. The iconic businessman's phone is the blackberry, a phone which has been dubbed the "Crackberry" due to its addictiveness.

Phones like the blackberry permanently connect professionals to their work. Spouses of people who are addicted to their phones go through stress as well. It is difficult to maintain a relationship with someone who cannot put down their phone or leave their work commitments at the office. It is ironic that cell phones were intended to help relieve stress, but in the end only increase it. Surprisingly enough, the computer and outlets such as email have little to no effect on workplace stress. This is because they do not provide immediate, fast access, and for the most part are used for a specific task. Cell phones, iPhones, and Blackberries all remove the user's ability to separate him or herself from the workplace. Wherever you go, your phone is with you and ready to receive texts and calls.

Top 5:
Sources of Stress

What causes our stress? In an annual survey by the American Psychological Association, here are the top sources of stress, and the percentage of respondents who identified each as a "very significant" source of stress.

1 Money	**76%**
2 Work	**70%**
3 The economy	**66%**
4 Family responsibilities	**59%**
5 Relationships	**55%**

Source: APA Stress in America survey, 2010 (most recent stats available)

Next, lets discuss health effects that can stem from social media addiction. When addicted to social media, people often lose sleep, or ignore basic needs in favor of their media account. Have you ever found yourself in bed for hours constantly refreshing your twitter/Facebook feed? This is a common way people lose track of time, or forget to do important tasks and work assignments. Originally, internet/social media "addiction" was thought of as a joke. How can anyone become addicted to an intangible concept? In recent years, it has been definitively found that people can become addicted to twitter, Facebook, or Instagram, and with negative affects.

How do we identify social media addiction? Social media addiction is most common in people who are diagnosed with depression. It becomes an outlet or distraction for a person's problems. Addiction occurs when a person feels like he/she needs to constantly have their phone in their hand, or feels like a status update/tweet NEEDS to be posted every few minutes. Anxiety issues can stem from social media addiction, which leads to high levels of stress. There are people who get very jumpy, nervous, or become unable to focus when separated from social media for too long of a period. Much like a hard drug, your twitter feed can consume your thoughts and your time.

Putting aside all of the physiological and health effects, can social media itself be directly harmful? The answer is, as you might have guessed, yes. The average person has around 250 Facebook friends. Chances are you will have a few negative interactions with people online. Someone could react negatively to a post you made, or you might not get the desired number of "likes" you were hoping for on your photo. When events such as these occur, questions begin to pop in your head. Am I not good enough? Did I not look pretty? Am I unpopular? The following hours can be consumed by thoughts such as these, and do not have a positive effect on you.

In the most unfortunate cases, I am sure you have heard of cases where people go as far as to take their own lives because they cannot handle the negativity or comments they received online.

So, how do we limit our time on social media, and assure that these effects do not happen to us? For many people, social media does not cause them any stress whatsoever. They can go about their day, checking their Facebook feed a few times a day, without putting much thought into it. For others, and people who might have addictive personalities, limiting time on twitter is not so easy. The best way to assure twitter or Facebook does not consume you is to have the two a day rule. Allow yourself to check and interact with social media twice a day, once at lunch and once before bed. Notice how I did not say to check it in the morning. When you check social media in the morning (usually in bed as you are waking up), you train your brain to "need" this fix.

A few years ago, I remember that when I forgot to put my phone on my nightstand before bed, I immediately got out of bed in the morning to find it. When my phone was on my nightstand, I laid in bed for another half hour or so browsing social networks. Deny your urges! It has been proven that people who make an active effort to limit social media in their lives end up being happier.

What about social media in the workplace? Many professional jobs force employees to sit at a desk or stay in a small area for most of the day. Employees can often turn to social media outlets and their phones to relieve boredom. While this is all well and good, this constant use of social media can result in anxiety and addiction. The more you use social media during the day, the more you begin to rely on it. Your brain feels bored, or feels as if it requires its media fix. As a result, it becomes difficult to focus on tasks and jobs you a trying to complete. The constant battle between resisting the urge to check your phone and trying to complete a task will result in amounts of stress on your brain and body. Symptoms can include fatigue, changes in appetite, loss of interest in hobbies, and consistently feeling bored.

Conclusively, social media can be a very good thing. It enables people to interact with each other, and for relatives to stay in touch over long distances. However, there is always a possibility of too much of a good thing. Too much social media can result in large amounts of stress and anxiety. As we previously discussed, it is possible to effectively limit your use of media. Be conscious of the time you spend on your phone, and instead of interacting with others online, see them in person!

Chapter 7: Guided Imagery

This relaxation technique is about imagining pleasant scenarios or experiences that can help calm the mind and body. It reinforces positive visions of oneself. However, it may be difficult to practice for those who often harbor intrusive thoughts. So, if you want to practice guided imagery, you need to be in control of your thoughts. Do your best to have positive thoughts.

Researchers have found that guided imagery is actually effective in reducing levels of stress. In a study that involved participants who practiced stress management techniques and guided imagery, it was found that their blood pressure has significantly gone down. In another similar study, the researchers have found that patients who practiced guided imagery were able to cope with their disease better than those who did not practice the relaxation technique.

Moreover, many other studies have shown that guided imagery is effective in reducing the levels of stress in patients with depression, post-traumatic stress disorder, and other mental health disorders.

Steps on How to Practice Guided Imagery

In order for this relaxation technique to work for you, you need to be in a peaceful environment. You can easily do this at home for as long as it is quiet and free from any distractions. If you intend to practice it regularly, you can even set-up a private space for yourself at home which is meant for this purpose.

Once you've found your ideal spot, you should settle yourself there. Sit on the ground or in a chair. Close your eyes as you keep your body relaxed. Start taking deep breaths.

When you are settled, you can begin the relaxation process. You have to select a setting. Imagine yourself doing your most favorite activity or staying in your most favorite place in the world. You can recall pleasant memories from your childhood. You can also create your own fantasy land.

Whatever you visualize, it has to be very personal and emotionally charged for you. It has to evoke positive feelings. Then again, if you do not have any particularly outstanding personal experience, you can simply imagine pleasant scenarios.

For example, you can imagine yourself relaxing at a beautiful beach resort or sitting in a cabin that is surrounded by trees and mountains. You can imagine yourself sitting near a waterfall or on top of a mountain. You can also visualize yourself in a temple.

Keep in mind that guided imagery is about relying on your senses. Hence, you should not merely imagine yourself in these wonderful locations. You should also pay close attention to the feelings that your imagination brings about. Wherever you are, you have to fully immerse yourself in it. Pay attention to your sense of sight, smell, taste, hearing, and touch.

Remain in this state of relaxation for as long as you want. Continue taking deep breaths. Do not allow intrusive thoughts to consume you. When you feel that you are ready to go back to reality, you should gradually prepare your body. Open your eyes slowly and begin to stand up from where you were seated. By this time, you should feel more relaxed, calm, and ready to face another day.

Chapter 8: Stress Management

Using Self-Help Techniques For Dealing With Stress

It may seem like there's nothing you can do about stress. The bills won't stop coming, there will never be more hours in the day, and your work and family responsibilities will always be demanding. But you have a lot more control than you might think. In fact, the simple realization that you're in control of your life is the foundation of managing stress. Stress management is all about taking charge: of your lifestyle, thoughts, emotions, and the way you deal with problems. No matter how stressful your life seems, there are steps you can take to relieve the pressure and regain control.

Why Is It So Important To Manage Stress?

If you're living with high levels of stress, you're putting your entire well-being at risk. Stress wreaks havoc on your emotional equilibrium, as well as your physical health. It narrows your ability to think clearly, function effectively, and enjoy life.

Effective stress management, on the other hand, helps you break the hold stress has on your life, so you can be happier, healthier, and more productive. The ultimate goal is a balanced life, with time for work, relationships, relaxation, and fun—and the resilience to hold up under pressure and meet challenges head on. But stress management is not one-size-fits-all. That's why it's important to experiment and find out what works best for you. The following stress management tips can help you do that.

Identify The Sources Of Stress In Your Life

Stress management starts with identifying the sources of stress in your life. This isn't as straightforward as it sounds. While it's easy to identify major stressors such as changing jobs, moving, or a going through a divorce, pinpointing the sources of chronic stress can be more complicated. It's all too easy to overlook how your own thoughts, feelings, and behaviors contribute to your everyday stress levels. Sure, you may know that you're constantly worried about work deadlines, but maybe it's your procrastination, rather than the actual job demands, that is causing the stress.

To identify your true sources of stress, look closely at your habits, attitude, and excuses:

• Do you explain away stress as temporary ("I just have a million things going on right now") even though you can't remember the last time you took a breather?

• Do you define stress as an integral part of your work or home life ("Things are always crazy around here") or as a part of your personality ("I have a lot of nervous energy, that's all")?

• Do you blame your stress on other people or outside events, or view it as entirely normal and unexceptional?

Until you accept responsibility for the role you play in creating or maintaining it, your stress level will remain outside your control.

Start a stress journal

A stress journal can help you identify the regular stressors in your life and the way you deal with them. Each time you feel stressed, keep track of it in your journal. As you keep a daily log, you will begin to see patterns and common themes. Write down:

• What caused your stress (make a guess if you're unsure)

• How you felt, both physically and emotionally

• How you acted in response

• What you did to make yourself feel better

Practice The 4 A's Of Stress Management

While stress is an automatic response from your nervous system, some stressors arise at predictable times: your commute to work, a meeting with your boss, or family gatherings, for example. When handling such predictable stressors, you can either change the situation or change your reaction. When deciding which option to choose in any given scenario, it's helpful to think of the four A's: avoid, alter, adapt, or accept.

The four A's – Avoid, Alter, Adapt & Accept

- Avoid Unnecessary Stress

It's not healthy to avoid a stressful situation that needs to be addressed, but you may be surprised by the number of stressors in your life that you can eliminate.

Learn how to say "no." Know your limits and stick to them. Whether in your personal or professional life, taking on more than you can handle is a surefire recipe for stress. Distinguish between the "shoulds" and the "musts" and when possible, say "no" to taking on too much.

Who stresses you out. If someone consistently causes stress in your life, limit the amount of time you spend with that person, or end the relationship.

Take control of your environment. If the evening news makes you anxious, turn off the TV. If traffic makes you tense, take a longer but less-traveled route. If going to the market is an unpleasant chore do your grocery shopping online.

Pare down your to-do list. Analyze your schedule, responsibilities, and daily tasks. If you've got too much on your plate, drop tasks that aren't truly necessary to the bottom of the list or eliminate them entirely.

- Alter The Situation

If you can't avoid a stressful situation, try to alter it. Often, this involves changing the way you communicate and operate in your daily life.

Express your feelings instead of bottling them up. If something or someone is bothering you, be more assertive and communicate your concerns in an open and respectful way. If you've got an exam to study for and your chatty roommate just got home, say up front that you only have five minutes to talk. If you don't voice your feelings, resentment will build and the stress will increase.

Be willing to compromise. When you ask someone to change their behavior, be willing to do the same. If you both are willing to bend at least a little, you'll have a good chance of finding a happy middle ground.

Create a balanced schedule. All work and no play is a recipe for burnout. Try to find a balance between work and family life, social activities and solitary pursuits, daily responsibilities and downtime.

- Adapt To The Stressor

If you can't change the stressor, change yourself. You can adapt to stressful situations and regain your sense of control by changing your expectations and attitude.

Reframe problems. Try to view stressful situations from a more positive perspective. Rather than fuming about a traffic jam, look at it as an opportunity to pause and regroup, listen to your favorite radio station, or enjoy some alone time.

Look at the big picture. Take perspective of the stressful situation. Ask yourself how important it will be in the long run. Will it matter in a month? A year? Is it really worth getting upset over? If the answer is no, focus your time and energy elsewhere.

Adjust your standards. Perfectionism is a major source of avoidable stress. Stop setting yourself up for failure by demanding perfection. Set reasonable standards for yourself and others, and learn to be okay with "good enough."

Practice gratitude. When stress is getting you down, take a moment to reflect on all the things you appreciate in your life, including your own positive qualities and gifts. This simple strategy can help you keep things in perspective.

- Accept The Things You Can't Change

Some sources of stress are unavoidable. You can't prevent or change stressors such as the death of a loved one, a serious illness, or a national recession. In such cases, the best way to cope with stress is to accept things as they are. Acceptance may be difficult, but in the long run, it's easier than railing against a situation you can't change.

Don't try to control the uncontrollable. Many things in life are beyond our control, particularly the behavior of other people. Rather than stressing out over them, focus on the things you can control such as the way you choose to react to problems.

Look for the upside. When facing major challenges, try to look at them as opportunities for personal growth. If your own poor choices contributed to a stressful situation, reflect on them and learn from your mistakes.

Learn to forgive. Accept the fact that we live in an imperfect world and that people make mistakes. Let go of anger and resentments. Free yourself from negative energy by forgiving and moving on.

Share your feelings. Expressing what you're going through can be very cathartic, even if there's nothing you can do to alter the stressful situation. Talk to a trusted friend or make an appointment with a therapist.

Get Moving

When you're stressed, the last thing you probably feel like doing is getting up and exercising. But physical activity is a huge stress reliever—and you don't have to be an athlete or spend hours in a gym to experience the benefits. Exercise releases endorphins that make you feel good, and it can also serve as a valuable distraction from your daily worries.

While you'll get the most benefit from regularly exercising for 30 minutes or more, it's okay to build up your fitness level gradually. Even very small activities can add up over the course of a day. The first step is to get yourself up and moving. Here are some easy ways to incorporate exercise into your daily schedule:

- Put on some music and dance around

- Take your dog for a walk

- Walk or cycle to the grocery store

- Use, the stairs at home or work, rather than an elevator

- Park your car in the farthest spot in the lot and walk the rest of the way

- Pair up with an exercise partner and encourage each other as you work out

- Play ping-pong or an activity-based video game with your kids

The Stress-Busting Magic Of Mindful Rhythmic Exercise

While just about any form of physical activity can help burn away tension and stress, rhythmic activities are especially effective. Good choices include walking, running, swimming, dancing, cycling, Tai chi, and aerobics. But whatever you choose, make sure it's something you enjoy so you're more likely to stick with it.

While you're exercising, make a conscious effort to pay attention to your body and the physical (and sometimes emotional) sensations you experience as you're moving. Focus on coordinating your breathing with your movements, for example, or notice how the air or sunlight feels on your skin. Adding this mindfulness element will help you break out of the cycle of negative thoughts that often accompanies overwhelming stress.

Connect To Others

There is nothing more calming than spending quality time with another human being who makes you feel safe and understood. In fact, face-to-face interaction triggers a cascade of hormones that counteracts the body's defensive "fight-or-flight" response. It's nature's natural stress reliever (as an added bonus, it also helps stave off depression and anxiety). So make it a point to connect regularly—and in person—with family and friends.

Keep in mind that the people you talk to don't have to be able to fix your stress. They simply need to be good listeners. And try not to let worries about looking weak or being a burden keep you from opening up. The people who care about you will be flattered by your trust. It will only strengthen your bond.

Of course, it's not always realistic to have a pal close by to lean on when you feel overwhelmed by stress, but by building and maintaining a network of close friends you can improve your resiliency to life's stressors.

Tips for building relationships:

1. Reach out to a colleague at work

2. Help someone else by volunteering

3. Have lunch or coffee with a friend

4. Ask a loved one to check in with you regularly

5. Accompany someone to the movies or a concert

6. Call or email an old friend

7. Go for a walk with a workout buddy

8. Schedule a weekly dinner date

9. Meet new people by taking a class or joining a club

10. Confide in a clergy member, teacher, or sports coach

Make Time For Fun And Relaxation

Beyond a take-charge approach and a positive attitude, you can reduce stress in your life by carving out "me" time. Don't get so caught up in the hustle and bustle of life that you forget to take care of your own needs. Nurturing yourself is a necessity, not a luxury. If you regularly make time for fun and relaxation, you'll be in a better place to handle life's stressors.

Set aside leisure time. Include rest and relaxation in your daily schedule. Don't allow other obligations to encroach. This is your time to take a break from all responsibilities and recharge your batteries.

Do something you enjoy every day. Make time for leisure activities that bring you joy, whether it be stargazing, playing the piano, or working on your bike.

Keep your sense of humor. This includes the ability to laugh at yourself. The act of laughing helps your body fight stress in a number of ways.

Take up a relaxation practice. Relaxation techniques such as yoga, meditation, and deep breathing activate the body's relaxation response, a state of restfulness that is the opposite of the fight or flight or mobilization stress response. As you learn and practice this techniques, your stress levels will decrease and your mind and body will become calm and centered.

Manage Your Time Better

Poor time management can cause a lot of stress. When you're stretched too thin and running behind, it's hard to stay calm and focused. Plus, you'll be tempted to avoid or cut back on all the healthy things you should be doing to keep stress in check, like socializing and getting enough sleep. The good news: there are things you can do to achieve a healthier work-life balance.

Don't over-commit yourself. Avoid scheduling things back-to-back or trying to fit too much into one day. All too often, we underestimate how long things will take.

Prioritize tasks. Make a list of tasks you have to do, and tackle them in order of importance. Do the high-priority items first. If you have something particularly unpleasant or stressful to do, get it over with early. The rest of your day will be more pleasant as a result.

Break projects into small steps. If a large project seems overwhelming, make a step-by-step plan. Focus on one manageable step at a time, rather than taking on everything at once.

Delegate responsibility. You don't have to do it all yourself, whether at home, school, or on the job. If other people can take care of the task, why not let them? Let go of the desire to control or oversee every little step. You'll be letting go of unnecessary stress in the process.

Maintain Balance With A Healthy Lifestyle

In addition to regular exercise, there are other healthy lifestyle choices that can increase your resistance to stress.

Eat a healthy diet. Well-nourished bodies are better prepared to cope with stress, so be mindful of what you eat. Start your day right with breakfast, and keep your energy up and your mind clear with balanced, nutritious meals throughout the day.

Reduce caffeine and sugar. The temporary "highs" caffeine and sugar provide often end with a crash in mood and energy. By reducing the amount of coffee, soft drinks, chocolate, and sugar snacks in your diet, you'll feel more relaxed, and you'll sleep better.

Avoid alcohol, cigarettes, and drugs. Self-medicating with alcohol or drugs may provide an easy escape from stress, but the relief is only temporary. Don't avoid or mask the issue at hand; deal with problems head on and with a clear mind.

Get enough sleep. Adequate sleep fuels your mind, as well as your body. Feeling tired will increase your stress because it may cause you to think irrationally.

Learn To Relieve Stress In The Moment

When you're frazzled by your morning commute, stuck in a stressful meeting at work, or fried from another argument with your spouse, you need a way to manage your stress levels right now. That's where quick stress relief comes in.

The fastest way to reduce stress is by taking a deep breath and using your senses—what you see, hear, taste, and touch—or through a soothing movement. By viewi ng a favorite photo, smelling a specific scent, listening to a favorite piece of music, tasting a piece of gum, or hugging a pet, for example, you can quickly relax and focus yourself. Of course, not everyone responds to each sensory experience in the same way. The key to quick stress relief is to experiment and discover the unique sensory experiences that work best for you

Chapter 9: Looking At Stress Through The Life Cycle

Most written narratives about stress deal with it in a broad/general, scientific and medical approach to an individual regardless of age. Only a few or none at all see stress, its causes, signs, symptoms, and impact based on the life cycle or stages of life. Of course, the last stage which is death will not be included. The feeling of stress is impossible for a lifeless body.

There are 6 stages of life: (1) pre-birth or pregnancy; (2) birth/newborn to infancy or from 0-3 years of age; (3) childhood or from 4-12 years of age; (4) teenage years/adolescence or from 13-21 years of age; (5) adulthood; and (6) death. Using the gender lens, male and female human being is said to have different body reaction depending on the stressor. This is because according to recent studies emotional quotient of female continues to dominate male. It is only in emotional self-control where women failed to score higher, but there is no gender difference has been found according to an article of Lipman in Forbes.com.

Stage 1: Pre-birth or pregnancy. Written in my book entitled: Positive Parenting: Parenthood: What Makes You a Parent That Children Loves is that a child inside the mother's womb is also affected by the way a mother craves for food, complain about getting fat, feeling uneasy, feeling the pain and even in the course of constipation. A child inside a mother's womb can feel everything and anything a mother are experiencing, hence there are stressors on human pre-birth stage. How it is possible then?

Pregnancy is considered a stressor to a woman, the reason she becomes emotional. The issue of getting fat, fear, and difficulty of pregnancy itself are the causes of stress for a mother and not for a child. It is the feeling of being emotional that becomes the stressor to a child inside the womb. This means that the stressor of a mother is not the stressor of a child inside the womb, but the effects of stress itself to a mother. Likewise, the nutrients from the mother's food are the one causing stress when it affects the baby's health inside the womb. Any changes in the body system of a mother can be a potential stressor to a child inside the womb then.

The impact of stress on a child during pregnancy may not be immediately visible except for those mothers who are alcoholic/drug dependent and smokers. Alcohol and smoking can produce birth defects. High level of stress during pregnancy can affect the child after birth, it could be on the emotional quotient, behavior and cognitive skills.

Stage 2: Infancy or 0 – 3 years of age. A fragile stage of life, a stage when a child starts to learn everything, from speaking, crawling, walking and distinguishing things around him/her. The fact that a child cry means the child is experiencing stress. Crying is part of a child growing up and that it is good for the heart. Excessive crying is called colic. Colic is excessive crying for no apparent reason. While there is no medical disorder condition currently attached to colic, it is still stressful for the child and of course to the mother or nanny.

What causes stress to a child at this stage are sensitivity to food or milk, losing mother's attention, presence of unknown people around the child, getting tired, losing toys, feeling the pain and having a sickness. Following the American Psychological Association (APA) category of stress, infant stress can be acute and episodic acute. Chronic stress is possible for those babies with congenital diseases.

The impact of stress on an infant is not that alarming and can easily be managed or corrected. An infant crying when hungry or when the stomach is upset because of the milk or the food taken. Feeding a child and a dose of medicine can do the job. An infant cry when the sleeping environment seems not conducive or not being able to sleep, a lullaby from a mother can do the job. The exception to these is congenital diseases.

Stage 3: Childhood or 4-12 Years of Age. The stage of life where the learning curve of a person is starting to rise and where curiosity is relatively high. A child belonging to this age keeps on asking a question, what is stressful is to answer their never-ending questions. All mothers can relate to this. Children also have a high percentage of information retention. Since the learning curve during the childhood stage is at an accelerated phase, the visibility of the impact of stress is not immediate. Something a mother or parents need to watch. For instance, inducing more fear that is stressful can affect the child's level of confidence today and in the future. It is worthy to note that emotional stress among children is normally deep-seated.

It is at this level where the causes of stress started to increase. This is because the participation or intervention of external actors increases or a child begins to interact externally. Apart from siblings, a child begins interactions with schoolmates, relatives, and neighbors, friends or not. With Siblings, causes of stress are petty conflicts, rivalry with parent attention, toys, and bullying. Except with the parent's attention, the same are the common causes of stress with the neighbor and school mates. Stress from school work is more on episodic stress.

Children are naïve and pure, the impact of stress is not that threatening to a child except for stress from parent's divorce and death which can have long term effect on child development. Parent's comfort is nonetheless still the best approach for stress management up to this stage. Medicine and doctors are secondary except on congenital diseases.

Stage 4: Teenage Years/Adolescence or 13-21 years of age. This is the stage where the context of suicide and any untoward actions can happen if not mitigated or arrest at an early stage. Causes of stress for this stage mostly came from external factors such as friends, school mates, relationships and school performance. Family matters and members of the family are no longer the principal sources of stress. But this is also the stage where teenagers started to understand family problems and financial struggle. They understand the reason behind divorce among parents.

Teenagers, however, put a premium on integrity and personal development, creating a good impression is of paramount consideration. Humiliation is something a teenager will avoid. In fact, the impact of stress caused by humiliation can be long term and may even be fatal. Physical looks and attributes can also be a source of stress and may have an impact on a teenager's confidence level. Funny how one pimple in the face can be stressful sometimes.

Since this stage is prone to chronic stress and can be fatal, the need for medical interventions commenced. Counseling and medical treatment are advised to avoid committing untoward actions and occurrence of depression to some extent. Impact of stress can also be a long time if not mitigated or not arrested at the early stage. Other symptoms stress at this stage are isolation in both physical and social media, crying, overeating or not eating, oversleeping and skipping of classes.

Stage 5: Adulthood. The long list of causes of stress and diversity of symptoms can be found in this stage. It is in the adulthood stage where the pinnacle of stress can be found. Acute stress leads to diseases and peculiar symptoms while chronic stress can lead to depression and suicide. Individuals capacity to handle stress varies, depending on the age, experiences, and exposures to the stressor.

What makes this stage different from the preceding stage is the capacity of an adult individual to hide and the ability to manage stress on their own. It is not self-medication but the ability of an individual to find the inner strength to manage or cure stress. Others find a cure through music and arts. Others call it a rebirth, when they turn to faith and missionary, works to heal.

Stage 6: Death. The last stage of the life cycle is death, where stress no longer matter. The stress here resides to those left behind.

Stress in the Human Life Cycle

There are 6 stages of life: (1) pre-birth or pregnancy; (2) birth/newborn to infancy or from 0-3 years of age; (3) childhood or from 4-12 years of age; (4) teenage years/adolescence or from 13-21 years of age; (5) adulthood; and (6) death.

The stressor of a mother is not the stressor of a child inside the womb, but the effects of stress itself to a mother. The impact of stress on a child during pregnancy may not be immediately visible except for those mothers who are alcoholic/drug dependent and smokers.

Crying is part of a child growing up and it is good for the heart. Colic or prolong crying may not have a medical condition attached to it but prolong crying due to stress must be attended to.

The impact of stress on an infant is not alarming and can easily be managed or corrected. Chronic stress is possible for those babies with congenital diseases.

A child begins interactions with siblings, schoolmates and neighbor, friends or not. They are the principal sources of stress. Parent's comfort is nonetheless the best approach for stress management up to this stage. Medicine and doctors are secondary except on congenital diseases.

Adolescence is the stage that is prone to chronic stress, it is at this stage where the need for medical interventions commenced.

It is in the adulthood stage where the pinnacle of stress can be found. Acute stress leads to diseases and peculiar symptoms while chronic stress can lead to depression and suicide. Individuals capacity to handle stress varies, depending on the age, experiences, and exposures to the stressor.

Chapter 10: Contacts

"Surround yourself with people that reflect who you want to be and how you want to feel, energies are contagious."
Rachel Wolchin

It is possible to find examples of people who have become truly successful while at the same time operating in isolation; one needs to really search for such examples. The majority of people need others. If you associate with the people that you aspire to be like it lifts your game. They give you both inspiration and motivation. Contacts are able to create opportunities and point out the pitfalls that you may face as they have often already walked the path that you are just setting out upon.

If you listen to, or read the biographies of some of the world's really successful people their stories will be littered with examples of those who have helped them along the way. People who have inspired them, trained them and opened doors for them. It is essential that you start placing yourself in a position where you can interact with those that inspire you. Their advice will not only prove valuable in guiding you, but will at the same time help you increase your confidence.

If you do not already know any of the people that you feel would be able to help you along the road to success, then it is time to engage in some strategic networking. Depending on the field you have now chosen as your arena for success you can begin making moves to develop contacts that hopefully will eventually turn into friendships. There are as many different ways of doing this as there are arenas for success. If you want to move ahead in business, then perhaps you need to join a network group relating to your particular business and if you want to be a musician then there may be musical groups with whom you can get together. It is rare that someone should enter an area where there is not some form of group gathering that could benefit his or her ambitions.

Even if you feel that a networking group is not for you there will be other places that you can connect with people. Sports clubs, wine tasting groups or your local church are just some examples of places that will provide opportunities to interconnect with others. As long as you are open to meeting inspirational people and are always on the lookout for such mentors then it is only a matter of time before you find yourself beginning to associate with the type of people that will be beneficial to your goals.

Once you break into the right circles you will become exposed to all manner of advice, information sharing and guidance. Even if much of the information is already known to you, you are still exposing yourself to a world of interconnectedness which has served to open doors for so many of the most successful people in the world. If you are lucky some of the connections, you make will turn into genuine friendships. You do, after all, share a similar field of interest. Friendship is always a valuable resource and often successful people find themselves becoming quite isolated so it is always a good idea to foster relationships that may become invaluable pillars of support in times of difficulty.

With the explosion of social media that has taken place over the last twenty years there are now more means of networking than ever before. Organizations such as LinkedIn and Facebook have a huge following and offer their members a means of networking in a wide variety of specific groups. Social media has its place, but while it does provide an easily accessible and useful tool, it should be remembered that it is just that a tool. It is not a substitute for genuine connection and with time being such a precious commodity we all need to weigh up the amount of time we spend on the net. You will need to assess for yourself if your online time is genuinely taking you in the direction you have chosen or if it is simply devouring time and providing you with a pretense with which to avoid seeking out other ways to interconnect.

One very important aspect of success is that it provides us with a chance to do something for others. In all our endeavors to achieve success we should be looking for ways to give back and in the area of interconnectedness this is particularly important. We cannot expect relationships to develop if all we do is take. We need also to be aware of others and to look for chances to be useful to them in just the same way as they are helping us. Don't be mean or secretive with your contacts. Share them and always open the door for others in the same way you have had doors of opportunity opened for you. Give advice and help with problems wherever possible. It can be tempting to be guarded and protective of hard found contacts and information but sharing is far more likely to lead to possibilities such as joint ventures and information exchange than it is to create a stronger competitor.

The people around you are the people you have chosen so if they make you unhappy you have nobody to blame but yourself. If you are miserable, you will have difficulty showing love or passion for anything. Whether it be your personal life or your professional life, the people around you were chosen by you and are kept in your life by you. You drew them into your circle and you are responsible for keeping them within your circle. Make a conscious decision about the kind of people you want to be associated with and the goals you wish to achieve. Attract people into your circle who have the same goals and ambitions. Successful people are usually attracted to other successful people, hard worker to hard workers and mild mannered individuals to mild mannered individuals. You define who you want to attract, think about that and make a concerted effort to portray the characteristics you wish to see in your contacts.

Associate with people who can help you on your path to reach your goals and you never know, you may have something to offer them in return. Seek out associates who have drive and ambition and people who will push you to your limits. Contacts who encourage you and who offer constructive advice and criticism. These are the kinds of contact who truly want to see you succeed and will help you in any way, even if you don't like what they are saying, if you sit back and truly reflect on their criticism or advice, you will see that they have your best interest at heart. If this period of reflection reveals otherwise, it is time to reconsider your association.

You do get those kinds of people in the world who pretend they want to see you succeed but deep down they wish for you to fail. Train yourself to seek out these individuals and rid yourself of their hidden negativity. The old saying "it only takes one rotten apple to spoil the bunch" is so true in this case. You don't need someone like this raining on your parade and infecting those around you with negative thoughts in a hope that you might fail.

The phrase "it's not what you know but rather who you know" is imperative when selecting people with whom you wish to associate. Of course don't adjust your own values and morals to befriend someone who is unkind or ruthless, just because of who they are or who they know. Their true colors will be revealed and they will at the end of the day do more damage to your reputation and attempts at reaching your goal than they will do good. These kinds of people will manipulate you, promising you the world but will do nothing but bring you down. Associate with like-minded individuals who follow the same values and morals as you do and chances are they will help you in any way they can in order for you to reach success and your goals.

You are responsible for who you draw into your circle. If you are unhappy with who is in your circle, only you are responsible for keeping them there. Do a thorough clean out of your circle. Think long and hard on what kind of individuals you wish to associate with. If you are passionate and driven, someone who is laid back and perhaps a little lazy, is not really going to give you any drive or encouragement.

Chapter 11: Change The Stressful

Situation

You know the causes of your stress and have worked on not being bothered by the uncontrollable triggers, now you need to learn how you can alter these stressful situations. Often, you aren't able to completely avoid encountering a stressful situation, but you do have the power of altering it.

For instance, your older sibling is always demoralizing you and has seldom anything nice to say about you. You cannot avoid meeting them as you both live under the same roof, but you do have the option of altering this particular annoying situation.

Let us find out the techniques you can exercise for altering worrying and traumatic situations in your routine life.

Don't bottle up your feelings

Try to be expressive of your feelings and opinions instead of keeping them bottled inside you. Like in the situation mentioned above, you could open up to your sibling respectfully, but firmly and tell them that their behavior is disturbing you. If they can't be nice to you, they should stop talking to you. Most of the times, an assertive behavior shows your opponent that you aren't scared of them and have the potential to confidently stand up against them. This makes them reduce the intensity and frequency of their ridiculing behavior.

Improve your time management skills

Many people are stressed when they aren't able to manage their time efficiently. Poor management of time means that you are unable to do assigned tasks at the required time and this definitely leads up to stress. Therefore, to avoid experiencing a taxing situation, you need to plan better especially in assigning time for the different tasks you need to undertake.

Pre-plan all your activities scheduled for the day at least one day before and allocate a specific time for each activity. Make sure to wake up early, so you can start with the tasks as planned. Once you start finishing your chores on time, you will actually feel good and this will help you deal with stress that is due to inability to complete assigned tasks at the expected time.

Be prepared to compromise

To alter the stressful situations, you need to be ready to compromise and change your unyielding behaviors. For instance, if you are upset due to the marital problems, you and your spouse are having and you are always blaming your better-half for the issues, then it is time, you take a break from the blaming behavior and try to improve your own behavior. Compromising and making positive changes on your attitude is a great way to come out of situations that might trigger stress.

See the Bigger Picture

Another great tactic of altering stressful situations is by seeing the bigger picture. Try analyzing your future to find out whether or not the perturbing situation will hold any significance for you in the long run, say two months or maybe a year. If you think you won't find that situation disturbing in the future, then you need to stop becoming perturbed by it right now because worrying about that issue won't help you at all.

Reframe Your Problems

Modifying stressful events as per your convenience is extremely helpful, especially if you are able to reframe the stress stimulating situations. You need to start viewing your stress causing situations with an optimistic approach. A stressful situation isn't always bad, sometimes it can provide you with the necessary break your body and mind is seeking for a long time.

For instance, you aren't able to reach office on time due to traffic congestion and that is making you lose your patience. Instead of fretting about the situation that isn't in your control, you need to relax and calm your mind by tuning in to a radio station you enjoy. It will calm your mind and help you take a break from the tensions around you.

Chapter 12: Some Weird Ways Of Dealing With Stress

-Drink juice preferably orange juice

There are many studies proving the fact that vitamins play a major role relieving stress, especially vitamin C. Vitamin C is usually rich in fresh fruit juices. The reason why I prescribe my readers to have orange juice to quickly shed some unwanted stress is because of its tangy and energizing taste. Fresh fruit juices are also known to give a quick boost to our immune system, which also helps if lowering down stress.

-Ear Massage

Do you have a cat? Have you ever touched and massaged its ears? If not then you should give it a try and observe how it pleases your cat. The same applies to us humans as well. Next time you're really stressed out at work try to massage your ears for a few minutes and concentrate on how it brings down to the level of stress.

-Have playful things on your desk

Keeping things like toys and random objects that make you feel positive on your desk is also a good idea to remain stress free at work. Just before you're about to begin something important and stressful, grab a hold of one of those toys, play with it for a few minutes and then get back to work.

-Worry stone

This technique of getting rid of stress is one of my favorites. Keep a small smooth and shiny stone with you all the time. Your worry stone should be kept in pocket and used at stressful moments. By simply rubbing the stone with your fingers and tapping it can provide quick relief against stress build-ups. While tapping and rubbing the stone, it should be imagines that all your worries, problems and stress are being transferred from your body into that stone through your fingers.

-Do things extremely slowly at times

Sometimes doing things slowly can actually speed up your overall day at work. If you are doing something in a great hurry, try to pause yourself and then go about doing the task in a very slow manner. This "slow motion" will not affect your mind and it will continue to process at the same speed. This exercise will let you regain your composure and the chances are that you will successfully complete the task at hand. Remember that this slowing down should only be for a couple of minutes. Try to have your lunch at work extremely slowly tomorrow, thinking about every bite and chewing it in slow motion.

-Do some laughter yoga

Some people may term it as laughter therapy but no matter what you call it, it has numerous benefits in stress management. It is a simple exercise where you have to forget about everything and just put your concentration in laughing hard. Make sure that you do this exercise when you are alone so that others don't get disturbed.

-Explore the world

Nature has a very positive impact on stress and human attitude. People who live closer to the nature (hills and forests) are known to have a calmer personality. For all our urban readers I advise to visit different places during weekends. Being in the same place and stuck in routine work negatively impacts our thinking pattern.

-Take time out to clean your office/cubicle

It is a proven fact that clutter contributes to tension and stress. Keep your office or cubicle clean and tidy at all times and you will be amazed on the impacts this simple habit could bring. If no one is designated to clean your place then you should not leave it as it is.

Taking 10 – 15 minutes out from your daily routine for cleaning your place is as important as showing up for work. Many of us are unaware of the fact that an untidy and cluttered office is the silent reason behind your daily stress. Spare 10 – 15 minutes for this purpose at the start of your day. Before you settle down, make sure that you have all the files, paperwork, stationery and other things at their place.

-Talk to yourself

How you look at things and take up your daily tasks is important. We all talk to ourselves, some are so loud that it seems weird but we all do talk inside. This self-talk is very important and actually shapes up our attitude towards different things especially when we are at work. Try to replace the phrase "I can do it" with "I got to do it". You will be surprised on seeing the impact of how a single word can change the whole attitude towards work. You will also experience the positivity building up inside you through this simple technique.

-Go outside and walk on the grass

Even modern day doctors prescribe their patients to walk on the grass bare feet.

This exercise is known to improve eyesight, helps in stabilizing blood pressure and helps to tackle stress as well. Even walking for a minute or two on the grass can keep you up and running throughout the day.

Chapter 13: Stress And Money

I'm about to get BRUTALLY honest...not that I'm not normally honest. However, this time I'm going to call out something I've been doing to sabotage myself and something you've probably been doing too. And the reason I'm saying this out loud to the world is so that YOU don't do it yourself.

It's so simple to do. It's the least risk thing to do. It's what most people will tell you to do. And it's also THE dumbest thing to do in my opinion, which doesn't explain why I do it myself.

For awhile now, I've been putting all my efforts and focus on the wrong thing. I was zeroed in and laser-focused on the money. The cold hard cash. The dinero. Why? Because I wanted it. Not because I needed it, which isn't a problem in of itself. You can admit that you want money. It isn't a dirty word. In fact, I give you permission to want a ton of money and admit it to anyone who asks.

The issue comes in where my mind was concentrating more on the money instead of the service I was giving. And the thing of it is that the service I provide is the MONUMENTAL number one reason why I do what I do. It's the reason I come to work every day, hour to hour and share my experiences, my results and my progress- with YOU.

I want to make a significant impact in the world. I want others who have struggled to raise a family and bring home the bacon to know that they are a powerful FORCE to be reckoned with and respected. I want to be the source of inspiration for others, not someone who manipulates you into believing that you are stuck where you are and there are no off-ramps in your life. You don't have to just "get through" the hours of every long day.

I want to lead by example and show you that you can have ALL that you want in this life and more. Yes, everything! And these days, I don't think I have been doing a good enough job because my mind has scoped in on the money. The bank account digits. Trying to Whack-A-Mole my goals and then go after another. And another. Until I've exhausted every bit of effort that I have nothing of quality left to give. The irony of all that busy work is that it doesn't work.

That's because the mission MUST be about more than just the money. There must be a force of inspiration that drives you forward, propelling you into greatness. And that just can't happen when you're worried more about cold green paper than you are about people. So it's no surprise to me that even though I'm crushing my goals, it hasn't been with as much excitement or profit as it usually is. I know I am tripping myself up.

I didn't get into the business of helping other to become a gazillionaire. The money is a bonus. It allows me to continue serving my purpose to motivate and inspire others to achieve their dreams. THAT'S why I show up every day. To stand in the middle of a crossroad and redirect traffic to the path that leads straight to victory. To show you that it is not only possible but that it can be probably when you program yourself for success.

It isn't enough to sit on the sidelines watching the events of your life go by. You must show up each and every day. Sunrise to sunset your actions must reflect your purpose. Here's a reality that's rarely pointed out. You make a difference either way. Whether you do something with your life or you don't do something, there are consequences to every choice and every action and inaction in your life. Do you want to advance the years not having any control over the effect you have on others? Do you want to allow the events and choices of others dictate your purpose? Or do you want to take the reins and ride your life to a place unsurpassed by most. To live a life most dream about and few ever realize?

You deserve a GREAT life. And while that may carry a different definition for each person, it still gives the same result. Happiness.

I want you to know that you can have it ALL and I want to show you that you don't have to be scared trying to go after it. Everything you've ever wanted has always been within your grasp and all you have to do is extend your hand and take it. Clinch down and hold onto it FOREVER.

I know I make a difference in people's lives. I know I help them everyday. But I struggle with the notion that I haven't been helping them enough. I want to increase my efforts and exponentiate the successful outcomes of people so that like a ripple in a lake, it extends far beyond the point of origin forever. And I want that for you too. I want you to wake up each day knowing you have the power to move mountains, to command the seas to obey you and to tame even the wildest beasts in your world.

I'm nobody of particular importance. Just a servant delivering a message. I can encourage you, motivate you and give you accountability. But what I can never be is YOU. There was only one job opening created in that position in the history of the world and only you can embody it.

All you need in order to be that employee of the month in the CEO of your own life is show up every day and be the best part of you that you can deliver. Show up, speak the truth, make a difference, make money and serve others. The more you do it, the more momentum you build and the more of an impact (and money) your will make in this world.

It really is simple. I have kicked myself in the ass for not keeping my focus and staying on track, being in alignment with my message. It happens. And it's important you know that. But what's more important is how you recover from that. The sooner you identify it and reset your focus, the faster you will find yourself on the right track again.

And when you're on the right track, that's when you can help the most people. And that's when you also make the most money. It isn't about the money, it's about the mission. But to be able to share your mission and serve, you need the money to sustain you. They go hand-in-hand so never apologize for accumulating your wealth. It simply serves as a vehicle to help more people.

We all have a message whether we think we do or not. We all struggle to find our purpose on Earth. We want to serve others and lead a rewarding life, but many times we don't know how. I would say in response to that that the first step is to never stop giving a damn. About friends. About family. About a higher calling. About each other.

Your mission is to put others ahead of yourself. Never stop thinking about serving them. Your loved ones. Your community. Always ask yourself how you can continue serving them. What can you share? How can you help? What can I give? The money will come but the impact you have is priceless.

Stop believing that you must struggle in life. I used to believe this. I used to believe that to struggle meant virtue. That I was more virtuous in God's eyes. More deserving. More humble. It's a lie. Struggling helps no one. It creates poverty and dependency on others. It does not serve a greater purpose than yourself and you cannot help anyone if you are struggling. It's a choice. Like most everything else in our lives. We can choose to struggle or not. It's not anyone else's fault but yours. You can blame it on whomever you'd like but the truth is that you are ultimately responsible for your situation. This buck stops with you.

If you're exhausted from struggling and you want to stop, then make that decision and STOP. Right this moment. Right this second. Just stop. Take the required steps you need to do something different. To choose a different path. No more victim status for you. Hand in your card and start working for your right to earn your financial freedom.

I know it's possible for you to succeed. I know this because I was exactly where you are right this second. I know because I've been through a lot of the same scenarios you're most likely walking through right now. In this very second, I've been there before.

And I am standing here telling you that there is another way for you. You ARE worthy of having it all and NOT settling for what you don't want in this life. No waiting your turn is required. It's within reach and always has been. You have a duty to impact others with your message and to reap the wealth of riches that can help you do so much more than you could do alone.

The time to begin is right now.

START your life. Start giving back and crazy, outlandish ways that align with your financial freedom. Don't be afraid to charge what you're worth and don't be afraid to DOMINATE your life. There are souls who CRAVE to hear your message. So many of them need your influence in their lives. And you're going to deny them that why? Because of fear? Because you aren't sure how to help? Because you feel like your skills/talents/experience aren't enough?

I don't have the secrets to the universe. But what I DO know is this- WE NEED YOU. And when you arrive and give us all of your essence, and deeply care about us too, the money POURS in. The struggle is no longer REAL.

A life mission and financial freedom go hand-in-hand. The sooner you begin your mission and influence the lives of others, that's when you will make headway with your income. The more you impact others, the more your income.

And it all begins with you answering "present" when the teacher of life calls your name. Say what's true in your heart, show up and share your journey. Reach out and lift up others with your message and do that every day consistently with your programs, offerings and content.

Show up > Share > Sell > Influence > Financial Freedom

It doesn't take a Harvard degree, but it DOES take consistency and discipline. A word of warning though. If you aren't failing occasionally then that means you aren't really trying. So embrace your failures. Learn from them because that's all they are. Opportunities to learn and succeed next time. So stand up, straighten your clothing, put your chin out and confront the day determined to absolutely KILL IT!

Chapter 14: How Stress Affects The Body

Stress can have detrimental effects on the human body, as well as the human mind. The human body is designed to withstand stress, but sometimes the reaction that your body has isn't enough to fully fight off the negative effects of stress. Stress can affect your brain, heart, blood pressure, and cause bad headaches. The human body deals with stress by absorbing punishment, and sometimes that punishment becomes too much for the body to take. Stress can also cause physical ailments such as nausea, headaches, and back pain. Undergoing more stress than your body can handle can cause all of these things, and more.

Headaches caused by stress can be very serious. Migraine headaches are among some of the most painful headaches that a person can be afflicted with. Stress can cause people to have severe migraine headaches on a regular basis. Migraines can cause people to have severe pain, nausea, vomiting, and sensitivity to light. Stress is one of the most common triggers for migraine headaches, and doctors really aren't even sure why. Something as subtle as a change in a person's hormones can be enough stress on the person to cause a migraine. Stress comes in many forms, so it is important to understand that some stressors have serious health side effects. Migraine headaches can be one of those unpleasant side effects.

Stress can actually do a lot of damage to asthma patients. The body can become quite endangered by an abundance of stressors, and asthma is no uncommon disease. Asthma is the restriction of the airways in a person's lungs, and sometimes stress can be a nasty asthma attack trigger. Asthma patients' bodies can fight against themselves in a stressful situation. In a stressful situation, the human body tends to speed up. Stress can make a person's heart beat fast, and as a result, they will start to breathe heavier and faster. This can be a harmful situation for someone who has asthma. Someone with asthma trying to take in too much air could start to hyperventilate, and they could pass out from lack of oxygen. Suffering from asthma can be very difficult when dealing with a lot of stress.

Diabetes is a disease in which the patient suffers from high blood sugar levels. These high levels can cause an arrangement of different problems. There are two types of diabetes, one in which the body doesn't produce enough insulin, and another in which the body doesn't produce insulin correctly or react to insulin correctly. How stress fits into the picture is tricky. Some people's bodies will actually alter their metabolism in times of high stress. Their bodies could start to produce insulin incorrectly, or stop producing it altogether if they suffer from diabetes. Stress affects someone with diabetes by directly altering their body's production of insulin.

Stress can also have negative effects on a person's heart. Heart problems caused by stress are all too common. Dealing with low to moderate stress on a long term basis can increase your chances for having a heart attack. When stress is left uncontrolled you are more likely to develop heart disease or high blood pressure. Heart attacks are among the most deadly health problems that you could have, and the more stress a person is exposed to could increase the chance that they have a heart attack. Stress can physically alter the way blood clots inside your arteries. This puts people at risk of heart attack. Of course, everyone's body deals with stress in a different way. That is why it is important to keep an eye on the way your heart and body react to the stressors that you encounter on a daily basis.

Our bodies are built to withstand stress, and even use it to our advantage in times of distress. This reaction physically changes our bodies. The body undergoes a chemical reaction when facing a stressful situation. The changes that the human body makes in times of stress are actually to protect it, but the severity of the stressful situation may make these changes take a toll on the body. Whenever a human is dealing with a stressful situation, these changes take place instantaneously. Rapid heart rate, quickening breathing, and even higher blood pressure are the ways your body physically prepares itself to withstand stress.

The affects of stress on the body are plentiful. Stress even has physical symptoms of its own that can be noticed. The physical symptoms that are exhibited from someone who is dealing with large amounts of stress are dizziness, fatigue, aches and pains, muscle cramps, upset stomach, and even indigestion. These are all physical ailments that can be cause by stress alone. That is why people will sometimes refer to stress as "the silent killer". You don't realize how much damage is being caused by stress, because it is nearly impossible to be able to tell if stress is causing the physical ailments that you are suffering from.

The human body is affected by stress in a multitude of ways, and even in a few ways that disguise the culprit being stress. Even though stress is a normal reaction to our perception of the dangers of change, it can still have a devastating effect on the human body. Nearly half of all people develop a stress related illness, at some point in their adult life. That number is increasing steadily as we learn more about stress, as well. Many people feel symptoms like lack of energy, body aches, headaches, chest pain, increased heart rate, and upset stomach as a type of flu. Little do many people know stress can actually cause all of these symptoms, and make your body less resilient to flu and cold viruses. Living a stressful life can increase your chances of getting sick, as well as take its own toll on your body.

Protecting your body against the negative effects of stress is no easy task. Doctors have been trying to figure out how to lessen the effects of stress on our bodies for centuries, and the only way to stop stress from ailing our bodies is to life a generally stress free lifestyle. But is living a stress free lifestyle even possible? Many people think that it is not. Living completely stress free would require a life of zero hardships, and that is frankly impossible. Everyone deals with change throughout their life, and the adjustment to this change is the very definition of stress. In order to live a stress free life, one would have to have the perfect living situation that requires zero change. That is why stress affects everyone on Earth.

Chapter 15: Eat Healthy Foods

Food is the fuel and the source of nourishment for the body, an integral part of our general wellbeing and good health.

It is important that we eat the right foods and eat well for us to be stay healthy. A healthy body is able to fend off the side effects of stress with ease.

Food and stress are uniquely interwoven; when faced with adversity some people have a sudden craving for food while others will lose their appetite. It is therefore necessary that we know the right foods to eat especially when we are under some sort of stress.

When we encounter stress we crave comfort foods such as fats and sugars. These foods are not healthy and cause harm to us and will cause us more stress.

To stay healthy and manage stress we have to avoid:

· Consumption of a lot of fast foods because they are unhealthy and more expensive than cooking for yourself, in the long run.

· Skipping meals because it is a catalyst for stress. If you miss meals you are likely to be fatigued and less nourished thus susceptible to stress.

· Too much caffeinated drinks which interfere with your sleep and deny you adequate rest.

· Eating wrong food types; eat a balanced diet and resist the temptation of eating too much of foods rich in fats and sugars. These foods only lead to weight gain and cardio vascular problems.

A poor diet will leave you with problems of hormonal imbalance and weigh problems – either loss or too much gain. You will develop a weak immune system and are likely to be susceptible to illnesses.

Unhealthy eating will also lead to imbalance of the blood sugar which may lead to diabetes.

Stress makes your body burn nutrients you consume much faster than normal that is why you should be on a healthy diet. It is wise that you replenish these nutrients to help cope with stress.

Work-life Balance

All work with no play makes Jack a dull boy! This old saying is very true; you need to have some time away from your job to have fun and engage in things that excite you and pump your blood.

Most adults who are stressed can trace the source to their work place because we spend a lot of time on the job. It is therefore important to balance the time we spend working and time for ourselves for a healthier lifestyle.

Work-life balance is about of dividing your time effectively and adequately between work and your private life. If you let work consume most of your time you and neglect or shortchange your personal needs you are will end up stressed.

When your personal life is in order, you are less likely to be stressed since you will worry less. Your mind will not be stretched from being divided between what you need to do at work and the personal matters awaiting your attention.

Spend time with family and friends; it is relaxing and healthy for you. When was the last time you went cycling or shopping with your children? These mundane activities are foundation to a well balanced healthy life devoid of stress.

If your private life brings you happiness you will ably face pressures that come your way.

After spending time with your loved ones, you need to set aside personal time for things that are self gratifying. Go for a massage or run a few laps at the neighborhood field, volunteer your services for a worthy cause etc. Such acts are great for boosting your emotionally wellbeing.

If you embrace a healthy work-life balance you will reap the many benefits. Personal nourishment and care is important for overall health.

Balance your private and professional life for a stress free healthy life where you are happier and revitalized.

Write; Pick Up Your Pen And Paper

Another technique of dealing with stress is writing; it is especially encouraged when one is so stressed or depressed. Putting down your experience, feelings and thoughts in a journal is very therapeutic for recovery and for defeating stress.

Writing works by clarifying your mind and thoughts and it is a form of therapy in the sense that it compels you to recall events and thoughts of the day on paper to give you a better avenue to analyze and understand what happened. It is also meditative; it slows down your heart as you focus on your writing to stream out your thoughts to paper.

Writing sharpens and stimulates brain functioning and activity to improve your mental acuity and concentration as well as improving your vocabulary. You are therefore better equipped to handle stressful situations.

When you write regularly, the stress triggers in your head are disrupted allowing you to better relax and sleep better. You get up well rested and energized. Writing also fights anger by removing the thoughts from your mind to the writing pad, essentially offering you a platform to vent it out.

When you write down your worries and problems it is easier to solve them; writing allows you to identify what the problem is, think it through over time and most likely come up with a great unrushed solution and avert the stress that you may have.

Having a to do list or schedule helps you focus and get organized , you are able to plan in advance to avoid last minute rushes or procrastinations that will only serve to make your life stressful.

Writing will boost your immune system; by slowing your breathing you are able to breathe in more oxygen to better nourish the brain and blood leading to faster healing and an enhanced ability to fight pathogens. Better breathing also strengthens the lungs, which has a positive effect in fighting respiratory conditions like asthma.

To reap the benefits of writing for better health and stress relief, it does not matter what you write, the main thing is to be able to jot down your thoughts and review them. You do not have to be a John Grisham! Write down what is on your mind because the healing power lies in you letting out the negative thoughts that are weighing on your mind.

Chapter 16: Healthy Stress Relievers

Taking a more positive approach when dealing with stressful situations can certainly help, but at the same time, you also need to nurture a healthy mental state in order to successfully do this. Drinking and smoking are not exactly the best things to do when you are feeling the pressure for they can actually cloud your judgment, further impairing you from doing what is right. So, what other outlets can you try when it comes to releasing negative energy brought on by stress?

Here are some examples you might want to consider:

- Relax and recharge. Go for a walk or a jog.

- Spend some time in nature and take a few days off.

- Go out with a good friend after work. A good laugh always helps.

- Sweat out all of that tension in your muscle at the gym.

- Buy yourself a punching a bag and take your frustration out on it.

- Take a long, warm bath. Make use of aromatherapy!

- Pick up a new hobby or continue one that you have stopped.

- Listen to music as loud as you want to and drown out everything else.

- Watch a feel good movie. Even if it brings you to tears, you will still feel really great about yourself and the world as a whole after.

-Get a massage! There is a proven link between stress and knotted up nerves in our bodies.

The point here is to distract and get your body moving so that your brain gets the jolt it needs. Stress can become a burden so great that it's almost paralyzing, leaving you struggling to find focus or even get out of bed. Another thing you can try is get really healthy -- make a complete lifestyle change if that is what's needed. Need some ideas? Check out the list below:

- Have a regular exercise routine. Physical activity has been proven to play a vital role when it comes to reducing the effects of stress, physically and mentally. If you make time for exercise, even if it is just 30 minutes a day and a few times each week, you will be able to release tension from your body and generate more calm.

- Eat healthier. The better nourished you are, the more capable you will be when it comes to dealing with stress. Any food that makes you feel lethargic can also increase the levels of stress in your body so try and avoid having these regularly. Also, make sure that you have a good breakfast and keep your energy up throughout the day by eating well-balanced meals.

- Reduce your sugar and caffeine intake. You may think that these help you deal with stress better, but the temporary highs produced by both of these will eventually lead to the dreaded sugar crash -- which can send your mood plummeting from 100 to zero within a few hours. Turn to something more natural such as fruit juice. You will also be able to sleep better and become less irritable. After all, many people end up having mood swings throughout the day just because they lack sleep. So make sure you get the full 8 hours!

- Avoid self-medicating just to feel relaxed. This would only offer you a temporary escape and relief to whatever might be stressing you out. Besides that, it can also be damaging to your health - both physical and mental. Do not mask the issue by taking medications when the real solution lies in facing everything head on.

- Always get enough sleep. Adequate sleep helps in fueling your mind along with your body while a lack of it can actually make you more prone to experiencing mood swings. People tend to be more irritable when they do not get enough sleep and

even the smallest things can tick them off.
So avoid all of that and make sure you get
the recommended 8 hours!

Chapter 17: Time Management

Techniques To Prevent Stress

In today's world, one of the most prevalent afflictions that people suffer from is stress.

Fast becoming a widespread lifestyle disorder, stress is a chronic illness that can affect your health in serious ways if left unchecked.

For those who are working professionals, deadlines and to-do lists are an everyday thing.

In order to manage stress levels and live a fit and healthy life, the one thing that can be done is time management.

A working and flexible schedule is the perfect way of combating spikes in stress levels.

In this section, we take a look at some of the time management techniques that one can use in order to reduce stress levels and live an enjoyable life.

Top Time Management Techniques to Manage Stress

There are a number of reasons that one should employ time management to prevent stress. Research has found that people who manage their time in an orderly and realistic fashion get more work done, are less stressed and have better quality of life. The best ways to manage time in order to prevent stress are:

1. Figuring Out Priorities:

The first step towards managing stress levels is setting your priorities straight. If you are someone who finds himself battling extensive to-do lists every day, it might be time to sit yourself down and figure some important details out. Ask yourself what your priorities are and whether the work that you are doing will help you achieve your goals. While deadlines are a part of any job, working towards something that you do not enjoy will most likely increase your stress level and decrease your overall work output. It is for this reason that one should figure out what the most important things in his or her life are and work accordingly. Priorities will also ensure that you can divide your time fruitfully among different tasks and manage your levels of stress. Overall, being honest and true to your goals is the best way to ensure time management and prevent stress.

2. Making a Workable List:

The second step towards managing stress is to make a workable schedule. While some use the calendar, you can also make to-do lists if it suits you. The best way to make the list is by noting things down according to priorities. There are some tasks that will need your urgent attention and some that can be worked through later in the day. Making lists ensures that you are organised in a neat fashion and not frazzled by the work load. All in all, the priority rating is one of the surest ways to manage stress since you will be aware of your workload and capable of handling it in a systematic fashion.

3. Scheduling Breaks:

The one thing that many people in the corporate world tend to lose their sleep over is deadlines. While it is important to submit the work on time and in a competent manner, it is equally important to take scheduled breaks. The reason one should do this is not only to reduce stress but also to increase work productivity and overall focus. It is a well documented fact that those who take breaks from their busy work schedule get more work done and produce a better quality of work. This is because breaks help us focus in a more efficient manner and also reduce the overall stress related to the job. If you are in a job where deadlines are the norm, it might be a good idea to schedule short breaks through the day.

4. Delegating and Working Smarter:

It is a known fact that the higher your position in a company, the more your workload. Naturally, the stress levels are also bound to be at an all time high. In order to manage the stress by time management techniques, the one skill that you must develop is the ability to delegate. Managing the work load is crucial not only if you wish to live a healthier stress free life, but also to ensure that you have some sort of social world outside of your job. The principle here is to make sure that you are working smarter to meet deadlines instead of logging countless hours and not reaping the same benefits. From filing paperwork to responding to emails, there are many minor jobs that can be handled by a member of the staff instead of you alone. The most useful and practical time management technique for corporate professionals is delegation and an organised working scheme. At the end of the day, these two are the most important aspects of stress management and efficient working.

5. Working in a Workout or Yoga Session:

When it comes to time management techniques, one of the minor but important things that could be done is scheduling a yoga break or a mid-day workout session. Working professionals will find that the afternoon hours do not pose as big a rush as the morning or evening ones. In cases like this, it might be beneficial to schedule a workout in the office gym if you have access to one. According to countless medical journals exercise is a great form of relieving stress and increasing concentration and focusing skills. Furthermore, it is a good way to get over the mid-day slump that many of us suffer from. All in all, when it comes to reducing stress, making sure that we get both body and mind moving is a top priority.

Chapter 18: Watching What You Eat

You can also keep stress at bay by being careful with how you eat. Some eating habits only tend to make your stress problems worse. You can keep that from happening by:

17: Avoiding Sugary Foods

The truth is; when you eat something sugary, you are likely to show less physical symptoms of stress. This is probably why - according to Harvard Medical School - you may crave sugary foods when stressed and **"stress eat"**.

But, scientists have determined that in the long run, a high-sugar diet can cause inflammation in a part of your brain called the hippocampus. This inflammation can cause you to show physical symptoms of stress. Psychology today has also reported that high sugar consumption is linked to depression.

Furthermore, eating sugary foods can cause glucose spikes in your blood. This has the effect of heightening your mood. However, that spike quickly goes down because your body releases insulin to stabilize the sugar and your mood shifts to that of feeling "low." These mood swings can produce symptoms similar to those of stress or worsen them if they are present.

Instead of rushing to take foods that are high in sugar, you can opt to consume things like protein, whole grain carbohydrates, vegetables and fruits. If you do so, you will be helping your stress situation than if you do the opposite.

18: Avoiding Alcohol Or Caffeine

Alcohol and caffeine are arguably the most consumed legal drugs in the world. In fact, many people turn to alcohol and caffeine to deal with stress. However, taking them when stressed may worsen the symptoms.

Let us look at caffeine first. Caffeine is a known stimulant. Caffeine affects the body by triggering your body's "fight or flight" response. When your body perceives a threat such as a stressful situation, this is the response that is triggered. Therefore, it follows that when you take caffeine when you are stressed, you are in fact making the underlying stress problem worse.

Alcohol, on the other hand, affects your body's hormonal balance. It does this by affecting the glands that produce the hormones as well as the tissues targeted by those hormones. Once your body's hormonal balance is affected, it fails to cope with stress in a better way.

Also, alcohol triggers the release of cortisol. And as you already know, this hormone worsens your symptoms of stress.

Therefore, if you want to better manage your stress levels, it is vital that you minimize your intake or stay away from alcohol and/or caffeine.

19: Strictly Follow A Balanced Diet

Apart from the above, you can just do the right thing and simply subscribe to a balanced diet.

This is an often overlooked part of the ongoing war against stress, especially considering the busy schedules that we keep these days. Nonetheless, ignore it at your own peril.

Dr. Mathew J. Kuchan , Ph.D. says that a well-balanced diet helps create a strong foundation for your body to fend off stress. He further explains that a well-balanced diet reduces inflammation and oxidation and this goes a long way to help fight stress.

What is even more interesting is that a balanced diet helps with blood flow. And when blood flow is increased in the brain, stress is effectively reduced.

Now I cannot spend time showing you how you can prepare a healthy diet plan since that is out of the scope for this book. But there is a lot of information out there

on the web that can help you easily figure
it out.

Chapter 19: Practicing Positive Affirmations

"I am never good enough." "I am not cut out for this job." "I just don't have the skills to get things done." These are some examples of negative thoughts that most people replay in their heads again and again. What they don't realize is that these thoughts, even though they seem harmless, are already affecting their lives, hold them back from opportunities, diminishing their confidence, and causing them stress.

Our thoughts are so powerful that they can affect our mood, perspective in life, and confidence. "Research tells us that every thought and emotion creates a chemical reaction because it immediately changes our neurochemicals that affect our mental, physical, and spiritual health," says stress expert Dr. Kathleen Halls in her interview with The Huffington Post.

That's why it's important to practice using positive affirmations to help motivate you, make you feel that you're in control, and help you manage stress.

"All 'Iz' Well"

A few years ago I had the chance to watch the Bollywood comedy-drama film, "Three Idiots." It is a coming of age story of three best friends who met at one of the most prestigious engineering colleges in India. The film revolved around the stories of these characters and how they were able to finish their degree, survive the terrors of the college's director, "Virus," and become successful despite the stressful situations they were in—all thanks to Rancho's (the lead character) mantra "All 'iz' well." Since then, I've been using this affirmation whenever I feel pressured and it has helped calm my nerves so I can think clearly about what my next steps should be.

You too could use affirmations whenever you feel stressed or when you just woke up so that you've already set a positive mood at the start of the day. Your positive affirmation or mantra should be something that resonates with you to help you regain your self-control even in stressful situations. Here are a few affirmations you could use to manage stress:

"I am in control. I am letting go of my worries. I am letting go of stress."

"I see stressful situations as an opportunity to prove myself."

"I am limitless; I can do anything that I set my mind to."

"My life is more enjoyable whenever I am calm and at peace."

"I choose to be happy."

"I choose to stay calm even when under pressure."

"I can do this!"

"I enjoy doing what I'm doing; it gives me fulfillment."

"My colleagues look up to me."

"My boss wants me to grow and be better because he sees potential in me."

Chapter 20: Lifestyle Changes And Stress Management

In this chapter, we are going to discuss how lifestyle changes such as your diet, daily exercise, and sleep help to lower your stress. What you eat and when you eat, your physical fitness and your sleep quality – all affect your ability to cope with stress.

Stress lowering eating

For most of us, dietary habits are less than perfect. You are living a stressful life and don't have time to think about a diet plan. However, what you eat and how you eat your food contributes considerably to your ability to manage stress. Eating the wrong things or eating at the wrong times can increase your stress.

Feed your brain

Scientists have conducted various studies on how different foods affect our mental state and how food can increase or decrease stress in our life. Serotonin – a naturally occurring chemical regulates your mood. Changing serotonin levels in your brain radically change the way you feel when you are stressed. Just like any prescribed medication, foods can also change the serotonin levels in your brain.

Choose low-stress foods

Lower your stress by following the below food guidelines

Complex carb: Focus on eating complex carbs, such as brown rice, cereals, pasta, and potatoes. Complex carbs boost serotonin presence in the brain and help when you are feeling stressed. However, avoid eating an excessive amount of complex carb.

Avoid simple carb: Avoid simple carbs such as soda and candy. Sugary foods will give you instant energy, but you will feel edgy, irritated and stressed afterward.

Eat enough protein: Eat more fish, chicken and other lean meats. Foods rich in protein provide essential amino acids to repair brain cells and enhance mental function when feeling stressed. If you are a vegetarian, then eat vegetables, beans, seeds, nuts and fruits for protein.

Eat vegetables: Eat dark-green leafy vegetables, squash, beans, and carrots. Raw or cooked, vegetables provide your body with essential nutrients and important vitamins that are needed to fight the negative effects of stress.

Fruits: Fruits are a good source of minerals and vitamins. Fruits contain antioxidants and vitamin A, B, C and E. All of them are proven remedy against stress.

Get plenty of potassium: Low-fat milk, bananas, wheat germ, whole grains, and nuts all provide your body potassium. Potassium keeps your muscles relaxed when you feel stressed.

Stress-relieving foods

Oranges: Oranges are rich in vitamin C and help to lower stress.

Nuts: Nuts, especially almonds contain vitamin B2, vitamin E, zinc, magnesium and help lower stress.

Milk: Milk contains calcium, magnesium, and potassium. All are stress-regulating elements. Milk also helps produce serotonin because it contains tryptophan.

Broccoli: Broccoli contains vitamin B and rich with magnesium.

Fish: Most fish contain vitamin B and help boost serotonin production. Tuna and salmon are rich with omega-3, omega-3 help to regulate the adrenaline rush when stressed.

Exercise and stress reduction

Exercise keeps your body fit and helps you better cope with stress. Sustained activity and exercise can decrease your blood pressure, lower your heart rate and slow down your breathing – all three are signs of reduced stress and arousal. Exercise is an effective way to reversing your body's fight-or-flight response.

Relax your brain

When you exercise, your mood changes and you start to feel different. This difference is a psychological and physiological response to the fact that you are doing something good for your body. Exercise helps to produce endorphins in your body. Endorphin is a natural morphine and has a calming effect on your body when you are stressed. Exercise daily.

Exercising is not a lot of fun. It requires stretching, pulling, lifting, straining, sweating and after a long day's work nobody is looking forward to that. Integrate exercise into your life and work. Here are some simple ways you can introduce small bits of exercise/activity into your daily routine.

Park your car at the farthest corner of the parking lot and walk to the office or to the grocery store.

When watching TV, do some set-up, stretches, jumping jacks.

Whenever get a chance, walk, especially when you are feeling stressed.

Do things that you like: such as

Play a sport – racquetball, bowling, tennis, basketball, baseball anything

Favorite activity – bicycling, swimming, dancing, ice-skating, horseback riding or even rope-jumping.

Getting a good night's sleep and stress management

When you feel stress, you also feel tired. A stressful day wears you out, and you feel tired. However, one of the main reasons for feeling tired is not getting enough sleep at night. If you are not getting enough quality sleep, you are more vulnerable to stress. The secret of quality sleep is knowing how much sleep you need at night and what strategies you should follow.

Know how much sleep you need

Most people need about 7 to 8 hours of sleep every night. However, studies show 50% Americans sleeps less than that.

Develop a better sleep routine. Here are some tips for better sleep:

Get a comfortable bed: Use a mattress that is comfortable for you because you don't want to wake up with a sore back or neck in the morning. Choose a suitable bed or mattress.

Use your bedroom for only sleep and sex: Ideally, you should use your bedroom for only sex and sleep. But if you live in a smaller apartment, then use your bed only for sex and sleep.

Avoid heavy meals before sleep: Avoid fatty and rich foods before bedtime. They interfere with the digestive system and cause sleep problem.

Sleeping pills and alcohol: Drinking several glasses of alcohol will reduce the quality of sleep, and you may wake up the middle of the night feeling tried. Avoid sleeping pills because they are addictive.

Consuming caffeine: Don't consume caffeine before bed. Soda, chocolate, tea, and coffee contain caffeine.

Turn off the light and keep the heat down: Turn off the light for a comfortable sleep and keep your bedroom cool.

Chapter 21: Social Stress

Social stress is Relationships generally and in the environment with others. Depending on the evaluation concept of emotion, the concern arises when an individual perceives, they don't have the tools to deal with or manage the circumstance that is particular and assesses a scenario. Since the danger of an event can be adequate, an occasion that exceeds the capability does not have to happen to experience stress. There are three sorts of phobias. Life Events are described as abrupt, profound life changes that need somebody to adapt quickly (ex. Sexual attack, sudden harm). Chronic breeds are described as persistent events that require somebody to create adaptations within a protracted-time period (ex. Divorce, unemployment). Daily hassles are described as minor events that happen, which need adjustment during the day (ex. awful traffic (disagreements).

Which may place one under risk for developing a mental illness and physical 29; when Stress becomes persistent, one encounters psychological, behavioral, and physiological changes? People are social beings by nature, as they have a Basic desire to keep social connections and requirements. Thus, they find maintaining ties that are positive to be beneficial. Social relationships contribute to success and can provide nurturance feelings of inclusion. Anything that disrupts or threatens to disrupt their connections could lead to societal Stress. This may consist of low social standing in society or at specific classes, giving a speech, interviewing with prospective employers, caring for a child or partner having a chronic illness, meeting new people in a party, the threat of actual death of a loved one, divorce, and discrimination. Social stress can arise in the micro-environment (e.g., family ties) and macro-environment (e.g.(hierarchical social structure). Social stress is the kind of stressor that individuals influence individuals more intensely and experience in their everyday lives.

Definitions

Researchers specify phobias and stress in numerous ways. Wadman, Durkin, and Conti-Ramsden (2011) characterized social Stress as "the feelings of distress or stress that people may encounter in social circumstances, and the related tendency to prevent potentially stressful social situations." Ilfield (1977) defined societal issues as "conditions of daily social roles which are ordinarily considered problematic or undesirable." Dormann and Zapf (2004) identified societal problems as"a category of traits, events, events, or behaviors that are linked to physical or psychological strain, and that's somehow societal in character."

Measurement

Social stress is quantified through self-report questionnaires. Through protocols and different strategies, researchers can cause Stress at the lab.

Self-Reports

There are and psychosocial stress. Such self-report steps include the Evaluation of Negative Social Exchange, the Marital Adjustment Test, the Risky Families Questionnaire, the Holmes--Rahe Stress Inventory, the Trier Inventory for the Assessment of Persistent Stress, the Daily Stress Inventory, the Job Content Questionnaire, the Perceived Stress Scale, and the Stress and Adversity Inventory. Researchers can employ interview evaluations. The Life Events and Difficulties Schedule (LEDS) are among the most popular tools used in the study. The objective of the form of step is to push the player to elaborate in their stressful life events, instead of answering striking questions. The UCLA Life Stress Interview (LSI), which is much like the LEDs, comprises questions regarding romantic partners, nearest friendships along with other associations, and family relationships.

Induction

In rodent models, defeat and societal disruption are two anxieties that are conventional paradigms. Into a cage home, a rodent is introduced from the disruption paradigm rodents which have naturally established a hierarchy. The competitive "intruder" interrupts the social hierarchy, causing the inhabitants social stress. In the societal defeat paradigm, an aggressive "intruder" and yet another non-aggressive male rodent battle. In a human study, the Trier Social Stress Task (TSST) is utilized to induce Stress. From the TSST, participants have been advised they must prepare and give a speech about why they are a candidate for their job. The experimenter movies while they provide the language and inform the player, that a board of judges will evaluate that address. Following the speaking part, a math task that entails counting backward by increments is administered by the experimenter. The experimenter prompts them to begin if the player makes a mistake. The threat of evaluation is your stressor. Researchers can assess the stress response by evaluating pre-stress salivary cortisol levels and post-stress salivary cortisol levels. Other standard stress measures utilized at the TSST are self-report steps such as the State-Trait Stress Inventory and physiological steps like a heartbeat. Couples recognize Specific regions of conflict. The pair then pinpoints a few subjects to talk in the future in the experimentation (ex. financing, child-rearing). Couples are advised to go over the battle (s) for 10 minutes while being videotaped. Brouwer and Hogervorst (2014) made the Sing-a-Song Stress Evaluation (SSST) cause stress in the lab setting. After seeing Pictures with backrest, intervals are educated to sing a song is complete. Researchers discovered that skin conductance and heart rate are higher. Through the message period compared to prior ranges. Stress levels are similar to that.

Statistical Signs Of Stress In Massive Groups

An analytical index of stress Correlations and variance were suggested for the identification of Stress and utilized in finance and physiology. The investigation of disasters showed Its applicability for the identification of concern in classes. It had been analyzed from the stress period beyond the political and 2014 Ukrainian economic catastrophe. There has been a simultaneous gain in the entire correlation between the 19 significant public anxieties in the Ukrainian society (roughly 64 percent) and their statistical dispersion (by 29 percent) throughout the pre-crisis decades.

Mental Health

Research has demonstrated that Stress Increases the possibility of creating adverse health effects. One potential study requested more than fifteen hundred Finnish workers whether they had "significant difficulties with [they are] coworkers/superiors/inferiors throughout the past six weeks, five decades, before, or not." Info on suicides, hospitalizations because of suicidal behavior, psychosis, alcohol intoxication symptoms, and medication for psychiatric disorders were gathered from the registries of mortality and morbidity. People who experienced conflict at the office in the previous five years with managers or colleagues have been far more likely to be diagnosed with an illness.

Those individuals have been indicated by research about the LGB population Identify as LGB suffer from mental health disorders, such as mood disorders and substance abuse, in comparison to. Researchers deduce the LGB people's risk of mental health problems derives from their stressful surroundings. Minority groups can confront high levels of stigma, prejudice, and discrimination regularly, resulting in the evolution of mental health disorders.

Depression

The risk for developing depression Increases after undergoing Stress; before getting miserable, depressed people frequently experience societal loss. One study found that it had developed depression around three times more quickly. In populations, individuals with family and friends who criticize make requirements, and make tension and conflict often have symptoms. The battle between spouses leads to more Psychological distress and depressive symptoms, particularly for wives. In particular, married couples ' 10--25 times more at risk for developing depression. Social Stress is related to higher gastrointestinal symptoms. In 1 study, whites reported to their experiences of discrimination and depressive symptoms. Irrespective of race, people who believed perception had depressive symptoms.

Stress

The biological basis for stress disorders is rooted in the Activation of the stress reaction. Fear, that's the defining emotion of a stress disorder, occurs when a person perceives a scenario (a stressor) as threatening. This activates the stress reaction. It might activate if an individual has difficulty regulating this stress reaction. Stress can arise if something is threatening or if an exact stressor isn't present. This may result in the development of a stress disorder (panic attacks, social stress, OCD, etc..). Social stress disorder is described as the fear of being judged or assessed by other people, even though no such danger is present. Research shows a link between Stress, such as Traumatic life events and strains, and also the development of stress disorders. A study that analyzed a subpopulation of adults, both middle-aged and young, discovered that people who had diagnosed with a stress disorder in adulthood experienced sexual abuse. Kids who undergo issues, such as reduction, in addition to damage, are more vulnerable to developing stress disorders compared to children who didn't encounter stressors throughout adulthood.

Long-Term Consequences

Social stress may have Effects that persist or develop in maturity. One longitudinal study found that kids were far more likely to have a psychiatric illness (e.g., stress, manic, tumultuous, personality, and substance use disorders) in late adolescence and early adulthood if their parents revealed more maladaptive child-rearing behaviors (e.g., loud arguments between parents, verbal abuse, and difficulty controlling anger toward the child, lack of parental support or accessibility, and unpleasant punishment). Psychiatric ailments and child temperament didn't clarify this association. Studies have reported that the connections between children Stress within stress, suicide, and melancholy depression, antisocial behavior, the family surroundings, and aggressive, oppositional, and conduct.

Relapse And Recurrence

Social stress can exacerbate psychopathological Ailments and undermine recovery. For example, patients recovering from bipolar disorder or depression are likely to relapse if there's tension. Individuals with eating disorders are more likely to deteriorate whether their relatives are aggressive to create critical remarks, or are over-involved. In the same way, higher symptoms are shown by outpatients with schizophrenia or schizoaffective disorder when the person in their lifetime is crucial and is much more likely to relapse when Stress marks their relationships.

Regarding chemical abuse Report more significant cravings for cocaine after exposure to societal stressors. Traumatic life events and social issues may also activate the worsening of these symptoms of mental health ailments. It can grow to be inactive and more avoidant.

Physical Wellbeing

Research has discovered a connection between various stressors and aspects of wellbeing.

Mortality

A stressor, social standing, is a Strong Predictor of departure. In a study of over 1700 British civil servants, socioeconomic status (SES) was inversely associated with mortality. People who have the lowest SES have worse health outcomes and mortality rates that are increased compared to those with the SES. Other studies have replicated this connection between SES and mortality in a range of diseases, such as infectious, digestive, and respiratory diseases. A study analyzing the association between SES and death in the elderly found that education level, family income, and occupational prestige were related to reducing death in males. In women, however, just real household income has been associated with reduced mortality.

Similarly, societal stressors from the micro-environment can also be associated with increased mortality. A seminal longitudinal analysis of almost 7,000 people discovered that socially isolated individuals had a higher chance of dying from any other cause. The social support that can be described as "the relaxation, Support, and advice one receives via formal or casual contacts with groups or individuals," has been associated with physical health effects. Research indicates the frequency of interactions, and the three facets of social aid perceived social support can forecast mortality thirty months.

Morbidity

Social stress makes people sicker. Individuals that have fewer contacts are at risk of developing a disease, such as cardiovascular disease. The one's social standing her or he would be to get a cardiovascular, gastrointestinal, gastrointestinal, neoplastic renal or other chronic ailments. These hyperlinks aren't explained by other conventional risk factors like accessibility, health behaviors, age, gender, or race to healthcare. Researchers interviewed participants to find out if they were undergoing conflicts, close friends, and relatives. Then they exposed the participants to the common cold virus also discovered that participants who have conflict-ridden connections were twice more likely to come up with a cold compared to people with no societal stress. Social support, particularly concerning relief for socioeconomic migraines, is inversely associated with substantial morbidity. Research that explored social determinants of health in an urban slum in India discovered that social exclusion, stress, and lack of social support are significantly linked to disorders, such as hypertension, coronary heart disease, and diabetes.

Long-Term Consequences

Stress in youth can have Raising the chance of developing diseases in the future, Long-term effects. In Specific, adults that have been maltreated (mentally, physically, sexually Abused, or neglected) as kids report more disease results, such as stroke, Heart attack, diabetes, and hypertension, or even severity of these results. The Adverse Childhood Experiences Study (ACE) that comprises over seventeen Million adults discovered that there had been a 20% increase in chances for experiencing heart disease for every sort of familial stressor that is chronically experienced in youth, which wasn't because of risk factors that were normal for Heart ailments like demographics or hypertension.

Retrieval And Yet Another Ailment

Social stress has been connected to health effects. If there was connection negativity with their spouse when controlling for severity of illness and treatment, patients having end-stage renal disorder confronted an increased risk. Similarly were likely when they had moderate to severe strain to undergo another event. This finding remained after controlling for disease status, health behaviors, and demographics. In terms of HIV/AIDS, the development may affect the virus into the disease. Research reveals the HIV-positive men who have more adverse life events, social Stress, and lack of societal support advancement into a clinical AIDS diagnosis faster than HIV-positive males who don't have as substantial levels of societal stress. For HIV-positive females, that have contracted the HSV virus, Stress is a risk factor for esophageal herpes breakouts.

Physiology

Social stress Results in a variety of changes that mediate its connection to bodily health. In the brief term, the physiological modifications summarized below are elastic, as they empower the nervous system to deal much better. Dysregulation of manipulation within the long-term of these or those systems may be damaging to health.

Sympathetic Nervous System

The sympathetic nervous system (SNS) becomes activated in Reaction to stress. Sympathetic stimulation arouses the medulla of the medulla to secrete norepinephrine and epinephrine into the blood vessels, which eases the reaction. Perspiration improves, heart rate, and blood stress constrict to permit the heart to beat arteries resulting in tissues dilate, with the additional weight, and blood flow to portions of the human body for the flight or fight reaction declines. If demand continues in the long term, blood stress stays elevated, resulting in hypertension and hypertension, both precursors to illness. Lots of human and animal studies have verified that the risk for adverse health effects increases. Studies of rodents reveal that hypertension is caused by stress and atherosclerosis. Studies of anti-inflammatory primates demonstrate that arteries clog. Although humans can't be randomized to receive social Stress because of moral concerns, studies have yet proven that adverse social interactions characterized by battle cause an increase in blood stress and heart rate. Social stress originating from perceived daily discrimination can also be correlated with elevated levels of blood stress throughout daily and a scarcity of blood stress dipping during the nighttime.

Hypothalamic-Pituitary Adrenocortical Axis (Hpa)

The hypothalamus releases Corticotropin-releasing hormone (CRH), stimulating the anterior pituitary gland to release adrenocorticotropic hormone (ACTH). ACTH stimulates the adrenal gland. Social stress may lead by interrupting the HPA system or activating the HPA axis. There are quite a few studies that connect signs and Stress of a disrupted HPA axis; for example, monkey infants show prolonged responses after an event. In people Cortisol after having a standardized laboratory stressor compared to people with no abuse history. Children reveal higher morning cortisol levels compared to kids. Their HPA systems don't recuperate after social interaction with their caregiver. Over time kids show cortisol's output. They didn't consist of disease results Even though these studies point to some disrupted HPA system bookkeeping for the connection between health and stress. Nonetheless, an HPA response to stress is supposed to raise the possibility of exacerbating or creating diseases like hypertension, cancer, obesity, cardiovascular disease, and diabetes.

Infection

Inflammation is Fighting with ailments and repairing tissue that is damaged. Though inflammation is elastic, chronic action can give rise to adverse health effects, such as diabetes, hypertension, coronary heart disease, depression, hypertension, [and a few cancers. Research has elucidated a connection between different Social stressors and cytokines (the mark of inflammation). Persistent social stressors, like caring for a spouse with dementia, cause higher high levels of cytokine interleukin-6 (IL-6), whereas intense societal stress activities in the lab have been demonstrated to provoke increases in proinflammatory cytokines. Likewise, when confronted with the other kind of societal Stress, specifically societal, participants demonstrated improvements in IL-6 plus a soluble receptor for tumor necrosis factor-α Increases in inflammation can persist over time, as studies show that chronic connection stress has been connected to higher IL-6 manufacturing six months afterward and kids reared at a stressful family environment indicated by negligence and conflict often reveal elevated degrees of lipoic protein, a mark of IL-6, in adulthood.

Interactions Of Bodily Systems

There is evidence that the physiological One another's working effects. For example, cortical will have a suppressive influence on processes, and cytokines can also activate the HPA system. The sympathetic activity may also upregulate inflammatory activity. Given the connections among these physiological methods, societal Stress may also affect health indirectly through impacting a specific physiological system, which then affects a unique physiological system.

Social Stress At Work

And, as associations experience budget discounts, cutbacks Workforce reduction, it's not difficult to recognize that workplaces may be stressful. Most of us know that stress may result in a plethora of issues with our health and well-being, but we also are aware it is not possible to merely prevent all sources of Stress. Specific kinds of stress (i.e., concern linked to deadlines or challenging tasks) are tough to relieve because we can't only move deadlines or create difficult tasks simple, but other kinds of stress (i.e., societal Stress) could be addressed.

Social **Stress**

Social stressors are described as scenarios and behaviors, Social that is linked to mental and physical strain. **Examples of societal stressors include:**

Verbal aggression from clients or superiors

Co-worker battle

Negative group surroundings

Organizational politics

Unfair treatment

Social stressors' expertise May Lead to a bunch of Results that are oppositional to a number of the most desirable effects and behaviors. The cause of this is that societal stressors deplete our working tools (or our capacity to cope' with Stress). Research has explicitly revealed that social stressor mainly causes the following results:

Reduced Job Satisfaction

Higher turnover

Feelings of failure

Reduction of productivity (because of time spent coping with 'scenarios')

Diminished altruism and organizational citizenship behavior (i.e., assisting conduct in the office)

Reducing Social Stress

Even Though it is known that migraines are not Avoidable, the fantastic news is that: there are actions that may be taken to mitigate the effects of Stress. Below is a listing of these activities that can if dedicated to, reduce societal stress and the negative impacts related to it:

For pioneers: prevent feelings of unfair/unjust therapy by becoming conscious of your interactions. Attempt to be viewed as a fair leader (offer feedback to all, make yourself accessible), rather than pick favorites.

For everybody: help set standards against co-worker aggression. Bear in mind that not all kinds of battles are reduced (e.g., disagreements about how to accomplish a specific task). However, societal conflict is usually negative and will result in social Stress. Steer clear of social battle by making certain debates are based on jobs, not individuals.

For leaders and HR: when hiring new workers, frankly assess the existence of social stressors at the comparative job atmosphere. Research shows that heart self-evaluations play a part in how workers respond to the presence of migraines.

Core self-evaluations contain self-esteem Self-efficacy and psychological stability Controller. All these can be quantified Using evaluation tools.

Chapter 22: Ways To Reduce Stress And Anxiety

Once you determine your personal stressors and decide whether to eliminate, minimize, or cope with each stressor, you are ready to move on to the next stress management step. Psychologists have some practical suggestions for minimizing stress in your life. By incorporating a healthy mindset, cultivating certain habits, and incorporating stress-reducing activities into your daily routine, you will greatly lower the negative stress in your life.

Stress-Reducing Habits and Activities

Learn to say "no"
Do not overcommit yourself. It is ok to say no to certain activities that are good but not necessary to your personal goals.

Do something fun every day
Schedule time each day to do something you enjoy, even if it is just for 20-30

minutes. Whether that is crafting, playing a sport, practicing an instrument, or reading a book, doing something that you like each day will help counteract any negative stress you experienced that day.

Schedule in relaxation time
Try to leave open time slots in your schedule to allow for sufficient relaxation and down time.

Schedule in vacation time
Try to schedule in regular days off of work, in between holidays. Taking a longer vacation like 5-7 days in the spring or summer is another great way to relieve stress and avoid work burnout.

Prioritize Sleep
Make sure that you get at least 8 hrs of sleep each night. This will keep your body and mind healthy and will help you to have a balanced perspective during the day.

Exercise regularly

Try to exercise for 20 minutes each day or more. Raising your heart rate will not only burn calories but will boost your endorphins and help burn off stress.

Eat healthy foods
Avoid junk foods, carbs, and foods that are high in fat. Fruits, veggies, and whole grains are great options for helping you to feel your best.

Express your feelings
Talking to a friend or therapist, or writing in a journal are great ways to help express yourself. Self-expression is necessary for releasing the emotions and stress that have accumulated during the day.

Connect with other people
Schedule time to socialize and visit with friends on a regular basis. Expressing yourself and learning to see things from another point of view are effective at lowering stress.

Change your perspective
Commit to thinking positively. Pick out the

good in every situation. Try to see every opportunity as a chance for growth.

Have   reasonable   expectations
Avoid stressing yourself out by having unrealistic standards or expectations. Instead, try to set realistic and moderate goals for projects, for yourself, and for a given   situation.

Try   yoga
Yoga not only helps increase your strength and flexibility, but controlled breathing exercises can help lower your heart rate and   reduce   stress.

Schedule   solitude
Many individuals help lower their stress by incorporating meditation, prayer, and moments of silence into their daily routine.

Chapter 23: Effects And Symptoms Of Stress

We've had a look at the possible causes of stress so now let's have a look at the effects and symptoms of stress so that you can understand for yourself when and why you need to prevent stress and take control. Some people might state, "I need to be stressed". This is not strictly correct... as you don't "need" to be stressed, maybe you need some adrenaline pumping for you to perform physically or mentally at a higher level, but stress in itself is debilitating if it is not managed. Very, very few situations are ever apparent when stress can help. When you have adrenaline, endorphins, serotonin, oxytocin, neuro-adrenaline all pumping around your body you maybe in a fearful situation. Let's think of an example, maybe you're being chased by a tiger- this is a stressful situation and your body needs the adrenaline to run faster to escape a chasing tiger that is hunting you down. But stress (or rather the natural chemicals released to create or deal with stress), if you do not work it out of your system, can be limiting and absolutely debilitating.

What are the effects and symptoms of your stress?

When you are stressed do you suffer with a lack of sleep or tiredness, are you absolutely wired and hyperactive, or lethargic?

Maybe your heart races or feels as though it stops for a beat or two.

Does your breathing become erratic?

Notice, when you're stressed do you clench your fists, scrunch your toes up, grind or crunch your teeth?

Do you have tension in your muscles, perhaps in your neck, shoulders or forehead? Maybe you get headaches?

What are the effects and symptoms of **your** stress?

What is difference between stress and motivation?

Lots of people tell me that speaking in public, whether professionally (presentations etc) or privately (wedding speeches) causes them a huge amount of stress not only at the time, but during the preceding weeks and months. My question to these people is always, "is the 'motivation' to give a fantastic speech greater than the 'fear/ stress' of giving the speech".

Do you feel pressured (stressed) or motivated and inspired to do things?

When looking at the difference between stress and motivation, for example, if you need to overcome a fear of speaking in public and the associated stress this brings, you may feel stressed and yet you want to give that presentation (for example a wedding speech) but you do not 'have' to do that speech. The stress created might be 'bigger' than your motivation to speak and therefore as a result your nerves might limit the quality of your delivery. In this situation, stress is not a motivator however for someone else the motivation to deliver a good wedding speech may 'over-ride the stress of delivering it. The desire to do a great job **MUST** be greater than the fear of getting it wrong.

People mistakenly think that they have to be stressed to do something well or get something done. An example maybe when someone feels that they are better leaving a work project until the last minute rather than planning time through the weeks preceding the dead line. They may get it done last minute, however much less stress might occur if they had done the task earlier in time.

To re-cap:

Look at – and understand - why you're stressed, understand why you are stressed. Look at the effects and the symptoms of your stress.

As you think about day to day things, emotions are managed by the 'amygdala' within the brain. The amygdala is a tiny, almond sized and shaped, mass of neurons and electrons deep within the brain which controls your emotional state. It tells your brain how to respond to emotions whether they are true or false. By that I mean, you could be watching a scary movie and even though the werewolf in the scary movie is not real, you can still feel stressed, anxious, afraid, your heart may pump, your breathing may become short and pronounced, you may have sweaty palms, a dry mouth, your hands maybe white as your knuckles grip the chair arms. All these things ... yet the werewolf is not real. So, your thoughts, in this example a scary wolf, could have led to emotions being created which led to the brain processing physical reactions to cope with the situation (eg fight or flight response). This is something called PNI; Psycho- Neuro Immunology. PNI is the effect of your thoughts, whether conscious or subconscious, on your emotions and your physical reactions. Basically, it is your subconscious mind talking to your brain which in turn controls your immune system and your physiology. That is about as scientific as we are going to get here but there is plenty more about this on the internet.

Now let's take a look at some other minor and debilitating things that cause these effects and symptoms. Some of the symptoms that you experience maybe very minor, others could be absolutely debilitating. If left unchecked, these symptoms may develop to be many times worse than they need to be. The great news is that most of these symptoms can be prevented quite easily. Your blood pressure, sleep patterns (or lack of sleep), muscle fatigue; all of these things can be prevented and managed effectively, and all will be revealed later in this book. If not managed they can lead to all sorts of health problems that can affect your personal life, your finances, your work-life, your self-esteem, your emotional or mental well-being, or even your physical well-being. They can lead to not being able to use machinery, or drive or even have children. It can affect your love-life. All of these things can be prevented.

We've looked at the causes, effects and the symptoms of stress, next let's look at some easy to apply stress prevention techniques.

Conclusion

It is my hope that this book was able to explore the existence of stress, what it can do to you; and most importantly help you with the necessary tools for managing it. It is always a struggle when someone is suffering from stress and it is nothing to be ashamed of. What is important is finding the heart to reach out for help because if you don't then the consequences are completely undesirable. Detecting stress early and showing willingness and commitment to overcome it is very important. Don't allow yourself to be buried in pain and sorrow, when there is so much that can be done to improve your health and wellbeing. The book offered clear solutions and advice, and it is my hope that you will use the knowledge gained to help yourself and others in your life.

Many thanks for your support and I wish you a healthy, loving, peaceful, and happy life!

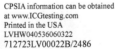